TRAUMA

TRAUMA

HEALING YOUR PAST
TO FIND FREEDOM NOW

PEDRAM SHOJAI, O.M.D.
AND NICK POLIZZI

HAY HOUSE, INC.
Carlsbad, California • New York City
London • Sydney • New Delhi

Published in the United States by: Hay House, Inc.: www.hayhouse.com®
Published in Australia by: Hay House Australia Pty. Ltd.: www.hayhouse
.com.au *Published in the United Kingdom by:* Hay House UK, Ltd.:
www.hayhouse.co.uk • *Published in India by:* Hay House Publishers India:
www.hayhouse.co.in

Indexer: Joan Shapiro
Cover design: Michelle Polizzi • *Interior design:* Nick C. Welch

The authors of this book do not dispense medical advice or prescribe the
use of any technique as a form of treatment for physical, emotional, or medical problems without the advice of a physician, either directly or indirectly.
The intent of the authors is only to offer information of a general nature to
help you in your quest for emotional, physical, and spiritual well-being. In
the event you use any of the information in this book for yourself, the authors and the publisher assume no responsibility for your actions.

Cataloging-in-Publication Data is on file with the Library of Congress

Hardcover ISBN: 978-1-4019-5902-9
E-book ISBN: 978-1-4019-5903-6
Audiobook ISBN: 978-1-4019-5954-8

10 9 8 7 6 5 4 3 2 1
1st edition, February 2021

Printed in the United States of America

For you, our reader.

CONTENTS

PREFACE

When we talked about writing a book on trauma, never could we have imagined we'd do it during the worst global pandemic since 1918, the most significant economic crisis since the Great Depression, the most wide-reaching race-related protests since the 1960s, and the most divisive political race for president in the U.S. in modern memory.

If the year 2020 had a theme, we're pretty sure it was trauma.

Like you, we find ourselves trying to navigate an unfamiliar, uncomfortable, and at times, downright terrifying world. We're all still finding our footing.

We won't pretend this book has all the answers to living through this moment, but we can tell you from the hundreds of stories we collected for this book, from our own lives, and from the trauma experts who have graciously shared their wisdom and insights into healing that you can resolve whatever pain you're going through.

While it may be hard to believe, no one says this moment in time has to become traumatic. As you're about to learn, the experts we spoke to were clear: *trauma is not about the experience that happens to us; it's what we do with it.*

We believe the insights and tools you're about to learn can help make this road a little easier and lighter.

If you take nothing from this book, please take this: trauma is not inevitable.

No matter what you experience during this time, it doesn't have to become traumatic. Painful? Sure. But you can work through that. You can learn how to release it before it gets stored in your mind and body. As much as this book is about showing you how to release your old traumas, it's also about helping you build your resiliency, so no matter what you face in life, you have the power, the tools, and the ability to process and integrate the experience.

The most painful experiences in our lives are often the catalysts propelling us toward even better, stronger, and more compassionate versions of ourselves. No matter what you're experiencing today, you can use it to transform your life—for the better.

Our greatest wish is that you use this moment to propel yourself toward greater self-love, more compassion for your neighbors, more meaningful relationships with your loved ones, and more peace in your world.

Stay courageous and strong.

— Pedram + Nick

INTRODUCTION

Trauma has a stranglehold on so many people, and they don't know it.

When you read the word *trauma*, what comes to mind? If answers like war, sexual abuse, physical assault, a car accident, post-traumatic stress disorder, natural disasters, or terrorist attacks popped up, you're not alone. But as you're going to learn, it is much broader, deeper, and more prevalent than you realize.

Trauma is unresolved pain.

It hums in the background of our lives, influencing our every thought, emotion, and action. It steals our life force; robs us of joy, faith, peace, and love; and gets in the way of successful professional lives. It prevents us from becoming the parents, spouses and partners, children, grandparents, sisters and brothers, friends and neighbors we know we can be. It causes our self-loathing, deep shame, and self-hatred. And it's the root of many unexplainable and often untreatable (from a Western medical perspective) illnesses, diseases, autoimmune disorders, and mental health issues like depression, anxiety, panic attacks, and suicide ideation.

When you live with trauma, it makes life in our modern, fast-paced, harried world that much harder. Consider for a moment, how often do you feel angry and verbally lash out at a co-worker or family members? How often do feel impatient and snap at your kids, spouse, partner, or employees? How often do people take advantage of your generosity or disrespect or exploit you? How often do you feel so exhausted that you can barely think straight or have the energy to power you through the day?

These reactions, and more, often come from trauma.

When you can't access feelings of joy, peace, calm, relaxation, clear-headedness, forgiveness, or love, then everyday stress overwhelms you. You shut down, becoming numb and desensitized to your experience of being human, to the people in your life, and the world around you. You don't have the mental, emotional, physical, or spiritual capacity to show up for your life or as the person you want to be.

This is no way to live. You can experience so much more.

It's possible. Thousands of people are doing it every day.

And in this book, we're going to help release you from your trauma trap so that you can do so.

WHAT TO EXPECT

Our mission in this world is to help people heal.

For more than two decades, both of us have worked in the health and wellness space. Nick as a documentary filmmaker, who's trekked around the world in search of ancient medicine and alternative healing modalities. He founded the Sacred Science website and blog to share the wisdom he's uncovered.

Pedram as an ordained priest of the Yellow Dragon Monastery in China, an acclaimed qigong master, master herbalist, and doctor of Oriental medicine, who helped thousands of patients in his Los Angeles clinic. He founded Well.org to bring more healing to people through movies, documentaries, and books.

Over the years, we've seen up close the unexplained illnesses, autoimmune diseases, depression, anxiety, strange digestive issues, migraines, brain fog, agonizing muscle pain, tension, and aches, and the utter exhaustion, failed relationships, addictions (to drugs, food, alcohol, sex), and unsatisfying professional lives that Western medicine has failed to heal.

Both of us are obsessed with the question *why*? We want answers, and nothing but the unvarnished truth. We were curious and needed to know why some people couldn't get better or heal their illnesses fully. What was blocking them, and what could be done to help them? The more experts we spoke to, the more we kept hearing about trauma and how unresolved pain often lay at the root.

Unfortunately, it's not something our Western society and medical establishment talks about as much as it needs to. That's partly because there is no pill to pop to make it disappear, nor is there a clear treatment plan that works for everyone. Treating trauma requires a more holistic, balanced approach that bridges the mental, emotional, physical, and spiritual bodies and often goes beyond what the Western medical establishment gets taught. It's a highly individualized process that frequently requires a multiprong approach combining some form of therapy, body work, and deep inner discovery along with lifestyle and self-nurturing practices.

It's also not something that happens after one therapy session—it's truly a journey.

Treating our inner wounds is also complicated because talking about trauma makes a lot of people wildly uncomfortable. Culturally, by and large it's not something we do. For many of us, admitting that we've been wounded by someone or some experience, whether buried deep in our past or recently, is hard to do. And sometimes the trauma we've faced can bring up feelings of shame and guilt, which can stop us from reaching out and getting the help we need—and deserve.

The more we dug into this subject, the more we realized it had to be the subject for our second book. Just like in our first book, *Exhausted*, we grabbed a camera crew and spent six months crisscrossing the U.S., interviewing more than 60 of the world's leading trauma experts. From therapists to healers to integrative medical practitioners to shamans to neuroendocrinology physicians to combat veterans to bodyworkers, we sought their wisdom into the harrowing and life-altering journey to heal trauma.

They graciously shared with us their knowledge, their personal stories and those of their patients (identities protected), and the best therapies, tools, and practices they use for themselves and teach to their patients.

Now, we share their collective wisdom and knowledge with you.

You will hear from experts like Dr. Margaret Paul, Dr. Joan Rosenberg, Dr. Keesha Ewers, Mary Morrissey, Dr. Patrick Gentempo, Brandy Gillmore, Andrew Marr, Dr. Carl Totton, Stacie Aamon Yeldell, Rabbi Arielle Hanien, Dr. Mark Gordon, and many more.

We've divided the book into two parts. In Part I, our goal is to help you better understand the true scope of trauma. There are a lot of misunderstandings and misperceptions, so we're pulling the rip cord on what it is; how it could be affecting your body, mind, and digestive system; and some of the less-talked-about sources from childhood, society, and religion. We can't heal what we don't see, and every chapter is filled with awakenings that will clarify what trauma is and where it came from, and help you shift your mindset about whatever you have experienced and the person you are today.

Then we roll into Part II, examining ways you can resolve your hidden pain, including the most common and effective therapies, ancient wisdom, natural remedies, and self-nurturing practices, and ways to experience self-love, set healthy boundaries, and find self-forgiveness. We want to arm you with the information and knowledge you need to make conscious choices about treatments and approaches that are right *for you*.

You aren't meant to use every therapy, technique, or tool that we share. No one does that. Instead, pick one or two that really resonate with and interest you. Build and add from there as you continue your quest to resolve trauma.

We've included some of the most powerful and effective treatments and tools that have helped at least hundreds of thousands of people release their pain and reclaim their lives. Even better, these techniques help build and strengthen your resiliency. If you can prevent trauma from getting in, you'll find more ease, joy, and peace in life.

Every chapter includes inspiring stories of people who have turned to face their inner shadows and painful pasts, and who have come out on the other side as stronger, happier, and more peaceful versions of themselves. We share what has worked for them on the *road to recovery*, the unique journey everyone must take.

At the end of each chapter, we've included *Reflections*, which will pose to you a series of questions designed to help you identify what— if anything—from that chapter needs follow-up. As you go through each chapter, we encourage you to note which, if any, topics strongly resonate with you. You can meditate or journal at the end of each chapter, or try to pay attention to your initial reaction as you're reading. Feel free to mark up this book or keep a separate journal so you can quickly write notes. By the end of the book, you're likely to have a list of areas to explore deeper on your own or with a trusted ally, such as a therapist or healer.

Lastly, we close every chapter with *Sage Wisdom*, which is an inspiring or thought-provoking quote from one of the experts we interviewed. You can also use these as prompts or during meditations. They're perfect for going deep within and reflecting on your trauma, life, and future.

While you can start with any chapter, we strongly encourage you to take the standard front-to-back approach. Part I will give you a strong foundation, shifting your mindset and perspective on trauma, your life, and your inner world. That's valuable information that will help you determine the right techniques and tools to start weaving into your life. Part II will give you specific suggestions on possible treatments and therapies that you can further explore.

If you've read our previous books and followed our work, you'll know that we're often direct and to the point. We call it as it is, and we're both tough-love kinds of guys who aim to inspire and encourage people to heal, expand, and develop to their fullest potential. Ninety-nine percent of the time, this style and tone works, but trauma is different. It requires deep compassion and patience mixed with a heavy dose of encouragement and lots of reassuring. We've intentionally toned down the kick-you-in-the-butt-to-inspire-you-to-greatness language that you will find in our other books and docuseries.

Also, we have to point out, this book is not about us. In our solo projects, and even in *Exhausted*, we often swung the camera around and shared stories and practices from our journeys too. Not this time. More so than any other project, we've stepped aside (i.e., stayed in our lane) to let the experts lead us along the path in *Trauma*.

THE PREP WORK

Resolving your trauma is quite possibly the most important journey of your lifetime. As you travel this road, you will uncover gifts, strengths, and talents you never knew you possessed. And you'll meet a version of yourself that will leave you in awe.

Before we set out on this expedition, we want to share a few mindsets and perspectives that can help make the trip easier.

Welcome trusted allies

No one heals their trauma alone. Everyone needs trusted allies. Admitting you need help and asking for it takes tremendous courage and strength. That's hard to do sometimes, yet it's so worth it. Every person who shared their story mentioned the support systems they had created. We're talking therapists and healers, doctors and energy workers, support groups and close friends.

Everyone needs help. No one gets through life on their own—*no one*. There are extraordinary people just waiting to assist you. Seek them out and let them into your life. Your life will change for the better when you allow these people into your world.

Especially in the early stages of your journey, this is so important. When we feel safe, we open up and release our trauma.

Imagine a new vision for your life

We're not talking creating a vision board with specific details. We're talking about seeing yourself in your mind's eye as a vibrant, healthy, peaceful person, living and loving life without trauma.

Just imagine yourself as someone who is healthier, happier, more confident, more relaxed, and more peaceful. You don't need to know what steps you'll take to reach this person. Just know they exist. Your path to them will reveal itself over time.

Be gentle. Be kind.

Working with our traumas can bring up very intense emotions and memories. Go easy on yourself. Give yourself a break. If a chapter seems too intense, stop reading. You can come back to it later. If necessary, seek support from those trusted allies we just mentioned.

For ourselves, not only do we make documentaries and write books together, we're also really good friends. Both of us know we can call the other anytime, anywhere, and talk about anything and everything—and we do.

You need these people, and you deserve them.

Self-nurturing and self-care practices (which we devote an entire chapter to) rarely come easily to us. We're taught to be hard and critical, judgmental, and harsh with ourselves.

Act the opposite. Ultimately, healing comes from finding self-love and reaching self-forgiveness. That takes practice and time (notice that theme?). The sooner you begin caring for yourself, the sooner you'll start releasing that stored pain.

See this as your hero/heroine's journey

We humans love stories, especially the hero/heroine's journey. That's when someone gets thrust out of their comfortable lives. They must venture into this unknown world filled with monsters, demons, and goblins. They meet allies and mentors who help them along the way. They stumble and trip; they get knocked down and beaten.

They hit the bottom where they're not sure they can keep going, but in the end, they defeat the mighty foe. They walk away victorious, and they've been changed.

Guess what? Resolving your trauma is the ultimate hero/heroine's journey.

The treasure at the end is *you*.

You will meet a version of yourself that you never knew existed. You will feel more *alive* than you thought possible. You will love and appreciate your life, your loved ones, and the world around you in ways you can't imagine. And you will unearth skills, talents, and gifts that you didn't realize you possessed.

Go on this quest. Free yourself from the trauma and find the treasure of a more caring, nurturing, and loving relationship with yourself that awaits.

YOUR JOURNEY STARTS *NOW*

Full disclosure: this isn't a how-to book that will magically resolve your trauma. Honestly, anyone claiming they can do that in a quick and easy five-step, one-and-done process is lying.

Releasing trauma takes *time*. Before you freak out, take a deep breath. This is a good thing. Every time you use a new therapy or therapist, embrace some ancient wisdom or a natural remedy, or give yourself a new self-nurturing practice, you let go of a little pain, which allows more light into your life.

Eventually, so much light will come in that it will overcome the darkness. Stick to the mantra: *Release pain, allow light. Release pain, allow light.* Be the tortoise and you will reach the finish line.

Not only will this approach help free you from the trauma, it will strengthen your *resiliency* muscle too. Resiliency is our ability to withstand whatever life throws to us. Two people may have the same experience, but one might walk away fine and the other might be traumatized. The difference lies within.

Keep in mind what all the experts told us: it's not the event that's traumatic; it's our response to it. You're going to hear us hit that point a lot—it's that important. The more we can process experiences in real time, the less likely they will go unresolved and get stored as pain. Growing up, most of us aren't taught how to do this. We have to learn it as adults, but millions of people are doing this every day and successfully releasing their trauma.

You are not alone.

Although both of us have devoted our lives to working in the alternative healing realm and could be labeled leaders in this space, we have our own traumas that need tending.

Pedram was born in Iran just before the revolution. His parents moved to the United States when he and his sister were just kids. They had fled the country and lost all their money. Like many immigrants, his folks aspired to give their children lives and opportunities they never could have found in their home country. Pedram grew up with an intense discipline and drive to succeed as a way to prove to himself that he not only belonged in America, but to show that his parents' sacrifices and hardships meant something. By and large, Pedram has succeeded and he loves the life he's created, but he's had to learn how to be kinder to himself, to not push and drive himself to the point of exhaustion. As you'll read in the next chapter, experts call this a "Little t" trauma.

He has to watch the voice inside his head that tells him he has to keep working hard and proving himself, he has to provide for his family, and he has to take full advantage of the opportunities his parents gave him with their sacrifices. That little voice formed when Pedram was just a kid—through no fault of his parents. It was Pedram's devotion to practicing meditation, mindfulness, qigong, and kung fu, and studying with true spiritual masters that made him aware this voice even existed. Even today, Pedram has to pay attention to his self-talk, to what's driving him, and to notice his thoughts and emotions so that it's not his traumas driving him.

For Nick, he's battled intense physical traumas that had left him with severe migraines that Western doctors had no idea how to treat. His pain led him to seek help and healing from shamans and medicine men in some of the most remote corners of the world. He studied, observed, and received extraordinary healing using ancient and indigenous techniques. He's come face to face with his pain while sitting through ayahuasca ceremonies in Peru and Native American sweat lodges. The healing he found using these alternative treatments inspired his documentary and book by the same name, *The Sacred Science*, which followed eight ill patients into the Amazon rainforest for healing. While his intention was to observe and document their experiences—and he did—he also discovered the shadows of trauma from his Catholic upbringing and unresolved self-worth issues born during his childhood and high school years.

More recently, Nick's learned he suffered a traumatic brain injury—he had no idea he had one—and has been working with a doctor who uses neurofeedback, meditation, and a heart-rate variability monitor to help retrain his nervous system. Even after all of these years in the alternative health world, Nick still has to focus and intentionally teach his nervous system to relax and must monitor his inner voice so that he doesn't constantly live in a state of fight or flight so that he can feel inner calm and peace throughout his day.

We share a little of our stories because everyone has their own trauma story. Everyone you meet in this world has experienced something painful—and the odds are they're still carrying it with them.

Both of us constantly work to acknowledge our traumas and to find ways to release them, because if we don't, they could get in the way of our business and life goals. More importantly, we know how easily unresolved traumas can get passed to children and how it can affect personalities and behaviors. We feel so connected to our life purpose to helping people heal, but the most important mission that we both share is to be great dads to our kids.

They inspire us every day to keep going, to be the best people we can possibly become. That means we have to look at our traumas, learn to accept them, and eventually release them.

Our aim in *Trauma* is to help you do the same. Our goal is to help remove some of the stigma, shame, and fear around this subject. None of us can change our pasts, but we can free ourselves from them so we can live as the best version of ourselves today.

That takes courage and strength, but we're willing to bet that you already have both in spades.

As you make your way through this book, be willing to look at your trauma as an observer. Be curious about where it came from. Be inspired by the stories of your fellow travelers and have faith that you can release your trauma too.

We believe that everyone has the power to change the course of their lives. We believe in the power you possess to heal.

We believe in you, so imagine us standing beside you right now. Together, we're shining the light of truth into the darkness.

Are you ready?

Your journey starts now.

PART I

UNDERSTANDING TRAUMA

CHAPTER 1

TRAUMA 101

Janelle's mom was very young when she got pregnant. When she gave birth to Janelle, she was only 17 years old, and she was terrified of being a mom. Janelle's mom never married her birth father, but when Janelle was two years old, she got married to another man. The man Janelle grew up calling "Dad" was emotionally and physically abusive, but only when Janelle's mom was at work.

The abuse continued until Janelle was 13, when her parents divorced. She felt relieved not to be around her father. But life was still hard. Janelle was a mixed-race kid (her mother was Caucasian; her birth father was African American), and she never felt like she fit in with her white or black friends. She had no community, no place to belong, and since Janelle's mom worked two jobs after the divorce, Janelle was often home alone.

Janelle didn't realize it, but these early experiences would ripple throughout time, impacting her self-esteem and marriage.

Annie was a military kid. By the age of 10, she had already been to eight different schools. The one in Florida was no different, except for one thing. Every so often, after saying the pledge of allegiance with her class, the loudspeaker would crackle to life. The school secretary would come on and ask Annie's teacher to send Annie to the vice principal's office. Annie's stomach would twist into a hard knot. She'd start sweating and her body would shake. Having no choice, she would go to the vice principal's office, where he would sexually abuse her.

Annie never said anything to anyone. She wasn't allowed. He told her if she did, he'd kill her, her parents and brother, and her dog too. Annie didn't even have the words to describe what had happened, so she kept the secret, burying it away, never to be remembered again.

From that moment, Annie became a perfectionist. She got into an Ivy League school, studied medicine (Western and Eastern), got married, had four children, and started a clinic. Annie seemed to have it all, until an autoimmune disease laid her flat and threatened to take away everything she had built.

On September 11, 2001, at 5 A.M., Bill clocked in for his shift as a network engineer at a huge telecommunications company in New York City. Televisions lined the room, attached to every pillar, to monitor what was happening in the area at all times. Bill loved his telecommunications job and co-workers and had been with the company for more than 10 years. Like any other morning, he began the day by fielding calls from customers—residential and commercial—troubleshooting and problem solving.

Then the first plane struck the World Trade Center. Images flashed across dozens of televisions, and Bill took calls from terrified people trapped in the towers, desperate to know what had happened and what they should do. Bill saw everything happening. He knew the truth and severity, and he wanted nothing more than to help the people on the other end of the line.

But there was nothing he could do for them.

Even though Bill wasn't at the World Trade Center that day, the images and cries for help haunted his waking and dreaming moments. The societal trauma he experienced was so real, the flashbacks so intense, that he took a leave of absence, hoping some time away from work would help him feel better and move on. It didn't work and the flashbacks kept coming, so he quit his job, broke his lease, and moved away from the city. For the next five years, Bill was haunted by the images, sounds, and utter chaos of that fateful day. He jumped from job to job, got into a string of failed relationships, and turned to alcohol to numb his pain and stop the memories.

OUR TRIALS

Janelle, Annie, and Bill have three different stories, yet everyone arrived at the same place: unresolved trauma that negatively affected their lives in very real ways.

As a society, we don't like to think or talk about trauma. It can make us feel uncomfortable. Pain and suffering are "negative," and we're taught "be happy," to "focus and think positive."

This isn't bad advice. Who doesn't want to feel happy and to experience a state of being that allows you to experience the richness and fullness of life and all its extraordinary gifts? We all aspire to experience true joy, love, connection, and wholeness.

But just thinking positive thoughts doesn't resolve our traumas. In fact, it can cause more damage. There are so many traumas that can leave a lasting imprint on us, even when we decide that we want to move on. We might slap a smile on our faces and look the part, but deep inside, we don't feel happy. We're pretending, and we know it.

Ignoring our traumas and pretending they no longer exist won't make them go away. They become ghosts in our closets just waiting to scare us.

"Trauma is a part of the fabric of reality," Stacie Aamon Yeldell, a board-certified music therapist, explained to us.[1] It is a part of life, and so many of us are walking the world, wounded. Research has found that over 70 percent of people have experienced at least one traumatic event in their lives, with about 30 percent having experienced four or more.[2]

Pause and really let that number sink in.

We're stunned. If we as a society and a culture are uncomfortable talking about trauma, pain, and suffering, how many people are actually getting treatment? How many people are seeking healing? How many people even believe they need healing?

Far too few. And that's a tragedy.

It's time for us to admit we have trauma that needs healing. As Dr. Patrick Gentempo, DC, told us, "My mentor, Dr. Nathaniel Branden, said, 'You can't leave a place that you've never been.' This was called the practice of self-acceptance. One time somebody said, 'Am I supposed to just accept that I have lousy self-esteem or accept whatever it is?' And he said, 'Yes, because until you do, you can never leave that place.'"[3]

Just as Dr. Gentempo's mentor explained, until we admit that we have unresolved traumas, we can never leave them either.

But when we do, we set ourselves on a course of healing that will forever change our lives. Our journeys to recovery and resiliency start by acknowledging that our traumas are real. In this chapter, we're focusing on what trauma is (spoiler: it's not the narrow definition that most people tend to think), the many causes of it, the difference between post-traumatic stress disorder (PTSD) and trauma, and the signs of it.

We know talking about and acknowledging this stuff is really tough. We also know that some of you may have to dig deep because your traumas have been covered and hidden for far too long—and that's okay.

We also know about the power of illumination. Shining a light into the darkness helps regain the power that our traumas have stolen from us. The first step in any journey is the hardest, *and* we know the bravery and courage that lies within you. Just be an observer in this chapter.

You've got this.

THE AWAKENINGS

Trauma Is Broader, Wider, and Deeper than You Realize

What is trauma?

All the experts we spoke with had a slightly different definition of it. From the over sixty trauma explanations we received, we condensed them into the following:

> Trauma is any event, experience, or situation that over-whelms our ability to cope and process what's happened to us. Whether it's a one-time event or something that happens repeatedly over time, the trauma becomes so deeply devastating and hurtful on a mental, emotional, physical, and/ or spiritual level that we lose a sense of ourselves. If trauma

goes unresolved, it can get stored in our systems—our bodies, minds, and nervous systems—causing long-lasting effects in our lives.

So, what causes this trauma that ruptures our well-being?

If rape, physical assault, experiencing a genocide or war, living through a natural disaster, or being in a terrible accident like a car crash came to mind first, you're not alone. Many people—ourselves included—immediately associate trauma with horrific experiences.

While that's true, it's not the full story. Every therapist, psychologist, psychotherapist, and healer we spoke with explained that trauma is far more wide-ranging than most people realize. They divided it into two categories:

- "Big T" traumas
- "Little t" traumas

Let's look closer at each.

"Big T" Traumas

"Big T" traumas are frightening, disturbing, and often life-threatening events. They can happen once or multiple times. Some of the most common forms of "Big T" traumas include:

- Sexual abuse
- Physical abuse
- Domestic violence
- Natural disasters
- War
- Accidents, physical trauma, or injury
- Death or loss of a child
- Mass shootings
- Witnessing a "Big T" event (watching anyone go through something horrific or tragic and not being able to control it)
- Experiencing a pandemic or other large societal event

"Little t" Traumas

"Little t" traumas are often prolonged, happen repeatedly, and are commonly dismissed. Some typical "Little t" traumas can include:

- Emotional abuse
- Developmental trauma (this occurs during childhood when we are still developing)
- Verbal abuse
- Childhood neglect
- Divorce
- Betrayal (such as being cheated on)
- Rejection
- Being shamed
- Death or loss of a loved one, including a pet
- Chronic stress and feeling overwhelmed
- Being bullied or harassed
- Experiencing a pandemic

"Little t" traumas are so varied and can seem so "minor" to us that we often don't realize the damage. For example, you could experience a "Little t" trauma when your boss says something that shames you during a staff meeting or you find out your wife has been having an affair.

Sometimes, it's the stacking of "Little t" traumas that cause damage. Brandy Gillmore, a mind, body, and energy expert with a Ph.D. in natural medicine, explained this concept perfectly. "If I have a little scratch on my arm, that's trauma to my skin. It's not the worst trauma in the world, and one little scratch might not be a big deal. But then you get twenty more little scratches, then thirty, then forty, and those start adding up."[4]

It's the adding up, as Brandy puts it, that eventually overwhelms our ability to cope with and process "Little t" traumas. As these traumas increase, they also affect how we manage our lives and experiences. They slowly wear us down, stealing our energy and peace of mind, so we have less resiliency when a large, often stressful event arises. "Little t" traumas can cause us to become impatient with our spouses, kids, co-workers, or direct reports. We may have little to no capacity to handle financial stresses, relationship issues, or health scares.

Life feels hard, because it is. And we can wind up with challenges in many areas of our lives. "We're under an enormous amount of stress with our lifestyles today," said Dr. Carl Totton, founder of the Taoist Institute and a licensed clinical and educational psychologist.[5] "The reason that we are reactive to that stress is because for years, we have accumulated all of these 'Little t' traumas that have added up, and it's like a barrel. Once the barrel gets full, then it begins to spill over. That spillage can result in symptoms including headaches, high blood pressure, diabetes, gut health issues, all of these conditions that are a system out of whack."[6]

Here's where it gets a little dicey. To some people, a "Little t" trauma can be experienced and felt as a "Big T" one, which leads us back to our earlier definition of trauma as anything that overwhelms our ability to cope. It disrupts our sense of feeling safe and okay.

Frankly, the breadth and depth of trauma (past and present) is staggering.

But before we fall into a bottomless pit of despair, there's hope. Yes, the list of what can be traumatic is long, but guess what? We're not alone. Most people have experienced trauma, and many have learned how to release it. We're connected by this shared experience, and knowing that makes us feel a little more compassion—compassion for our brothers and sisters who are in this journey with us.

It makes us realize, too, just how important it is to heal unresolved trauma and to build a solid inner foundation so we can remain resilient, no matter what trials and tribulations meet us on this journey of life.

Right now, the most important person in this trauma story is *you*. It's cliché, but true: you have to take care of and really love yourself first, before anyone else can.

Maybe you experienced a "Big T" trauma or multiple "Little t" events or some combination—chances are, you did. Whatever your trauma, please give yourself a moment of grace and acknowledge whatever experience may still be wedged in your heart, mind, body, or soul.

Your trauma was real, and it deserves to have a light shone on it and for you to eventually let it release its grip on your life.

All Trauma Matters

When we interviewed our trauma experts, we wanted them to dig into very specific types of traumas. Actually, we expected them to, but what we took away is: *all trauma matters*. Whether it's "Big T" or "Little t," it's about dealing with the trauma you've experienced so you can heal from it and move forward in your life.

When we compare traumas, we often judge them—and by extension ourselves. It can be easy to minimize "Little t" traumas. We convince ourselves "to suck it up. Don't be a whiny little brat. So what if Mom or Dad were hardly around? I had a 'normal' family; I'm fine."

In fact, you're far from fine. You may have grown up feeling unseen and unheard, unloved and abandoned by your caregivers, and these impacts can ripple across time. They may be manifesting as failed relationships with your children or spouse; trouble holding a steady job; feelings of dissatisfaction, discontent, and unhappiness; or serious health problems that no doctor can fix.

There is no "better" trauma or "less bad" trauma. Granted, there is an obvious road to recovery for someone who experienced a gunshot wound versus someone who has been bullied by their boss every day. But the point we are making is that it's all personal and it's all subjective to your own story.

On the other hand, we may misconstrue healing from the "Big T" traumas as weakness. We might tell ourselves, "Yes, I was raped in college" or "My husband beat me, but I survived. I've moved on. That stuff is in the past." While it's important to not let our past trauma define us, it's crucial to acknowledge it.

Trauma is trauma is trauma.

Whatever you've experienced matters, and it needs to be healed. Judging our trauma only leads us to judge ourselves, making our journeys to recovery and resiliency more difficult. Right now, we're not asking you to feel differently about your trauma. But for a moment, we invite you to see your trauma as neither big nor small, bad or less bad, painful or less painful.

Your trauma just *is*, and all trauma matters equally.

PTSD vs. Trauma: It's Not What You Think

It's easy to confuse trauma and PTSD, but they're different. You can have a traumatic event without experiencing PTSD. PTSD is considered a psychiatric disorder that can happen after experiencing or witnessing an extreme event such as a natural disaster, mass shooting, terrorist attack, violent assault, rape, or other dangerous and life-threatening event.[7]

When you suffer from PTSD, you may have intense and disturbing thoughts about the experience, including flashbacks or nightmares, and you may have very strong emotions around it so it feels like you keep reliving the moment in real time.[8]

As a society, we relate PTSD with war and our soldiers and veterans. But while soldiers do experience PTSD, they aren't the only ones.

In the United States, PTSD affects approximately 3.5 percent of the population, and 1 in 11 people will be diagnosed with PTSD at least once in their lifetime.[9] And consider this: a recent study found that parents of autistic children and those with a rare disease reported significantly more PTSD symptoms than parents of typical children.[10]

The American Psychiatric Association explains that symptoms fall into four categories:

1. Intrusive thoughts. This includes recurring memories, dreams, or flashbacks to the event that make the person feel like they're reliving the experience again.

2. Avoiding reminders. To prevent themselves from thinking about what happened, a person with PTSD may avoid other people, places, or things that could remind them.

3. Negative thoughts and feelings. This may include distorted beliefs about themselves and ongoing fear, shame, guilt, or blame. They may also stop doing the activities or hobbies they once enjoyed.

4. Arousal and reactive symptoms. This may include being irritable with angry outbursts, being reckless or engaging in self-destructive behaviors, being easily startled, or having trouble sleeping.[11]

For it to be PTSD, symptoms must occur for longer than one month. Why a month? Because after you've experienced a traumatic event or witnessed one, your system has to process it to integrate it. You're likely to find yourself thinking of the event or having flashbacks or unexpected emotions around it. You may dream about it. All of these reactions are very normal after an intense experience.

But if you were nodding your head to the symptoms and it has been months or years after an experience, then it could be a sign that you're having a more extreme reaction. There is nothing wrong with you, if that's the case. There's no shame here. It doesn't mean you're weak. Think of it as a clear signal that it's time to seek guided care from a trusted therapist and/or healer who can help you work through the experience.

Healing from PTSD is absolutely possible. We have heard extraordinary stories from people who have regained their lives and are living in ways they never thought possible. We're going to share some of these stories, and we're going to revisit this topic throughout the book.

Hang in there.

The Signs and Symptoms of Trauma Vary

It would be a lot simpler if the signs of trauma were clear. But they're not. They're as wide and varying as the causes for it. That's because as unique individuals, each of us responds to trauma differently. In fact, we may not experience symptoms for weeks, months, or even *years* after an event.

If you've experienced a "Big T" event, then it may be easier for you to connect the dots. But that's not always the case. Some people have blocked out their "Big T" experiences, and many "Little t" ones can remain hidden.

This may sound depressing, but there are a number of conditions and symptoms that the medical community *has* connected to trauma. So if you're not sure if an experience has disrupted you, consider if any of the symptoms plague you.

Some of the common signs include:

- Anxiety
- Depression
- Panic
- Deep feelings of shame and/or unworthiness
- Intense emotional outbursts—anger, denial, rage, sadness, nonstop crying
- Addictions
- Troubled relationships
- Unhappiness
- Feeling disconnected from yourself, people in your life, and the world
- PTSD
- Physical symptoms (including migraines, autoimmune diseases, muscle tightness, high or low blood pressure, and digestion issues like constipation or diarrhea)

There are several means to uncover the trauma that is impacting you. There is the ACE Quiz, which is a self-assessment tool that measures ten types of childhood trauma (acestoohigh.com/got -your-ace-score/). Many trained psychologists and therapists also screen for and assess for trauma, including PTSD. If you're considering working with someone (and we highly recommend you do), ask if they are a trauma-informed therapist. These therapists are trained to work with people suffering from a traumatic experience and typically approach their patients with a deep understanding of the mind-body connection and how unresolved trauma affects someone in many ways.

THE ROAD TO RECOVERY

Janelle, Annie, and Bill needed to address their underlying traumas if they had any chance of changing their lives for the better. Thankfully, they did. For each of them, their journeys began with admitting they needed help and that they had unresolved pain.

Interestingly, only Bill knew the connection immediately. At the urging of friends and family, he connected with a therapist who specialized in cognitive behavioral therapy (one of the most effective forms of treating PTSD). After completing a 16-week intensive program, Bill saw his life dramatically shift as his symptoms lessened. He's since gone on to explore other healing modalities that have helped him heal more. Today, Bill is in a long-term relationship with a woman who understands and supports him, and he's gone on to use his experience to help other people heal from their PTSD by becoming certified in different healing therapies.

For Janelle and Annie, it took more work to uncover their trauma roots.

After Annie learned she had an autoimmune disorder, she began to practice yoga and meditation more religiously. During one of her meditations, she saw herself as a young child, and her memories came flooding back. Because of her medical background, Annie immediately knew that she had started releasing trauma. While she had a lot of tools for healing, it wasn't a journey she could take alone.

Shortly after remembering what happened, she began working with a therapist trained in EMDR (eye movement desensitization reprogramming). Through diet, movement, meditation, and different therapeutic approaches, she eventually healed her trauma and her autoimmune disease.

It took many months for Janelle to find her traumas—in fact, she hadn't been looking for them. Janelle felt depressed, unhappy, and at a crossroad with her husband of more than 20 years, and she was looking for ways to save her marriage. They met when she was 19, and he was the first guy to show her attention. While he wasn't physically abusive, he was emotionally disconnected and distant. He rarely showed affection and never asked her about her day at the bank where she worked or told her "I love you."

Janelle felt like he didn't listen to her or care about her needs, and she didn't feel comfortable talking to him about them. And truthfully, she didn't think she deserved more.

A friend suggested Janelle see a psychoanalytic psychologist. For the first time in her life, Janelle felt heard and seen. Her therapist created a safe space for Janelle to understand how her past traumas were impacting how she showed up in her marriage.

Janelle's father's physical abuse was easy to spot and work on healing. The emotional abuse from him, the abandonment she felt from her mom, and the disconnection she felt from being a mixed-race child and having no real sense of community—these issues were harder to identify and work through. But as Janelle did, she saw how the traumas had piled up over her lifetime and how she had lived more than 40 years feeling abandoned, unlovable, unseen, and ignored.

Today, Janelle's much happier. She's expressed to her husband her desire to work on their relationship. He's been receptive and they're talking about seeing a marriage counselor together. She also wants to go to college and is planning to take night classes. There's still work to be done, but Janelle's trying to put herself first, acknowledge her needs and wants, and work to heal the wounds from her past.

REFLECTIONS

Take a few minutes and freewrite or meditate on what is jumping to the forefront for you. Did anything surprise you in this chapter? Did you learn anything about yourself? Did you pause at all? Many of us are quick to brush aside painful experiences, so consider if there may be an event, or multiple ones, that could be lodged within. If it helps, make a list of those moments so you can return to them later or use with a trusted ally to go deeper.

SAGE WISDOM

"I don't see trauma or symptoms of it as something that's wrong with us that needs to be fixed. It's about trying to reframe the trauma in a way that makes sense, and so we can understand that everything that happens to us in life actually moves us toward wholeness and a higher consciousness."

—Michael Mollura

CHAPTER 2

STORED IN THE MIND AND BODY

For more than 30 years, Sundar had experienced debilitating migraines that knocked him out of commission for days. Nothing that he did worked to make them stop.

Working as a registered nurse for a major hospital, he knew all the treatments. He took hot showers, drank caffeine, and rested in a dark, quiet room. His doctor had prescribed medication, and he'd take it, but it only sometimes worked.

The migraines started in college, and while he had learned to live with them, they had taken a heavy toll. He loved his job, his co-workers, and taking care of the patients on the cardiac floor. Most of his reviews were very positive, except for one area: sick time.

It used to be he'd get a few migraines a year, but the frequency had increased to at least once a month, and it was starting to impact his job and performance. Sundar's manager questioned him and made comments about how often he would leave a shift early or call out sick. "You provide excellent care, are very attentive to patients, and you're a leader on the floor, but I'm concerned that I can't rely or depend on you," Sundar's manager said one day. "I'm very concerned that your migraines and health are getting in the way of doing your job, and we need to find a better solution."

This terrified Sundar. He'd been to so many doctors and had so many brain scans, but they were all normal. He had tried yoga and meditation, and had been tested for food sensitivities and vitamin and mineral deficiencies. An herbalist had given him different tinctures and pills to try, including feverfew, willowbark, and ginger, and he had worked with a chiropractor. He needed this job, and he was doing everything he could to stay healthy and take care of himself, but *nothing* had worked and no one had answers.

Sundar felt like he was coming to an impasse: he would have to either quit his job or he'd get fired. Neither option was what he wanted, but he had no idea what to do next.

OUR TRIALS

We're masters at ignoring our traumas and convincing ourselves that we've moved on, when we really haven't.

"We tend to forget that it [trauma] even happened, which means that it's put out of sight and out of mind," explained Dr. Carl Totton.[1] "It's been said that 'time heals all wounds.' It's not true. Time conceals all wounds. That disordered energy doesn't go away. What you call the shadow, things that are disowned that we can't really integrate, it's put into the background in the subconscious. But what's in the background tends to come back and stab us if it hasn't been identified, addressed, and balanced."[2]

If we're not able to release the toxic experience of trauma, all that shock and pain gets internalized. This is the body's wisdom; it attempts to protect us from something horrible.

It may not be tomorrow or next week or next year, but eventually the burden of carrying that hidden trauma will become too heavy for us to bear. It manifests in unexplainable and untreatable physical aches, pains, ailments, and diseases.

Somewhere in your body, your trauma is stored. Maybe it's in your hip, lower back, or neck. Maybe it's revealing itself in anxiety, impatience, or hair-trigger anger. Maybe it's returned in numbness, where you don't feel anything, you don't feel grounded, and it's hard to be connected to your life, this world, and the people in it.

Trauma expresses itself differently in everyone. There are very real physiological explanations for whatever physical and/or mental health challenges you're facing. In this chapter, we're going to unpack what's going on inside your body and mind. During this leg of our journey, we'll look at what's happening to your nervous system during and after a traumatic experience. We'll show you some of the reasons why your mind may be holding on to a trauma, and some of the latest, most innovative research into the brain and its connection to inflammation, traumatic brain injuries, and PTSD.

It's our hope you can use this information to see whatever physical or mental struggles you may have differently. When we change our perception, we can change the course of our lives. We know how frustrating it is to live with chronic pain, an illness, or a mental health issue that no doctor can seem to treat or cure.

Your body and mind *want* to heal; they want to release the stored trauma that's interfering with the fullest expression of *you*. Joy. Happiness. Peace. Love. Wellness. Ease. Balance. Centeredness. Calm. Vitality. Health. This is our center; it's the core of who we are and who we're meant to be in this world.

Your body isn't broken and neither is your mind. It's the unresolved traumas that have thrown you off your center, but that center is still there, and it always will be. Your quest in this lifetime is to find your way back to it.

THE AWAKENINGS

The Body and Mind Connection Is Real

Your nervous system is the bridge between your mind and body.

It sends and receives countless messages from one to the other that will determine your body's responses. Think walking, talking, swallowing, blinking, chewing, moving your hands, wiggling your toes, breathing, and all the other actions and movements that happen that we're both conscious of (standing from a chair and walking to the kitchen for a glass of water) and unconscious of (breathing or swallowing).

Our nervous system operates in two states:

- *Parasympathetic*, also known as rest and digest, regulates digestion and elimination processes, energy recovery, and relaxation.

- *Sympathetic* controls our fight, flight, or freeze response during a perceived stressful or dangerous experience. Think of this as your defense system.

You can't be in both states at the same time. You switch into sympathetic (fight, flight, or freeze) mode when your internal alarm system, called the *amygdala*, senses danger. The amygdala sits in a part of the brain responsible for processing emotion and everything from sights to sounds to smells that you're exposed to.

When it senses a threat, it triggers your body's fear response by sending an "Alert! Danger!" message to your nervous system, which in turn flips into the sympathetic state. In this mode, the hormone adrenaline floods your system. Your heart races, your pupils dilate, and you sweat more. Your blood gets redirected from certain organs and processes like digestion to your extremities so you're prepared to fight, flee, or freeze. This is all normal and natural, and your body is doing what it was designed to.

Here's where our story goes sideways. In a perfect world, as soon as the threat passes, you would discharge, or release, all the excess energy that was created. You'd process your threatening experience and let it move through your body so that you could return to the parasympathetic rest-and-digest state.

You see this demonstrated in the wild. A lion will chase an antelope. It's running for its life, adrenaline coursing through its legs, senses heightened, and it escapes. Once it's no longer in danger, the antelope will start shaking, convulsing, and contorting its body. What looks like a seizure is actually the antelope discharging and shaking off its extra energy so it can move from the fight, flight, or freeze state back into the parasympathetic rest-and-digest mode.

In our modern world, we don't shake it out or process the experience. We ignore it, pretend it didn't happen, or convince ourselves we're over it. We can bury our past traumas in unhealthy behaviors.

And sometimes what we use to avoid and numb ourselves from our pain can turn into addictions, which cause even more harm to ourselves and the people we love.

Nothing we do will discharge the energy that was created, but it still has to go somewhere. That somewhere is in muscles, joints, tissues, and fascia in our necks, shoulders, hips, lower backs, and anywhere else our bodies can find to store it.

To be clear, that storing still doesn't make the trauma go away. Think of it as a giant boulder that gets dropped into a stream. The water doesn't go through the rock, it goes around it. Well, your body has to adapt and learn to go around this trauma boulder that's come out of nowhere.

Look at people's postures. You'll see some people who round their shoulders and upper backs in a defensive stance. Other people will pull back their shoulders, push out their chests, and assume an aggressive self-defense pose. These are the unique adaptations our bodies will make after we've experienced a trauma that goes unresolved.

As we adjust our bodies to work around the trauma, our natural structures and postures change and can lead to pain in our physical bodies. Think headaches, migraines, scoliosis, chronic lower back pain, knots in your neck or shoulders, and stiffness in your hips and joints.

You may also find that some muscles are very tender to the touch, like there are spots on your body that would hurt if someone poked you. You may flinch or feel a tingling sensation. These spots are signs you may be storing unresolved trauma and emotion.

Once this trauma has been stored, it's not going to just disappear. It takes work, often with someone in the healing community who will help guide your body to release what's stored. There are many ways to do this, which we'll chronicle in Part II.

For now, just know it's possible to heal, and many of the experts we spoke with had inspiring stories of people who have healed by releasing what's inside. Dr. Patrick Gentempo, DC, explained that over the last twenty years, he's noticed a pattern with his chiropractic patients. "Sometimes I adjust somebody and they immediately start crying. 'I don't know why I'm crying right now,' they'll say. Sometimes they start laughing. It's very spontaneous and a very large emotional response occurs because they've been storing something for a very long time that their body has welded off."[3]

Try scanning your body now. Take note of the aches and pains, soreness, or tenderness you have and where. Is there an old "injury" you've nursed, maybe something that's nagged you for years? Or is there what you'd call a weak spot, such as when you're really stressed or overwhelmed and you notice a crick in your neck or you get a stitch in your right side? If you can, try to note when you first noticed this pain, like "it started after the surprise 28th birthday party my friends threw me."

So many of us with trauma disassociate from our bodies. We are not used to paying close attention to how we feel in them. Regularly cataloging any physical aches, pains, and injuries will help improve our awareness. Learning how to tune in to your body can also come in handy when you start digging into trauma with a specialist, therapist, or healer.

There is such a connection between your mind and body. We don't need to hate our physical selves or our bodies' aches and pains. Your injuries, may in fact, be the stars in the night sky that can guide you toward healing and release.

Your Mind and Body Are Caught in Fight, Flight, or Freeze

Your nervous system was designed to flip back and forth between the parasympathetic and sympathetic states. The fear-based fight, flight, or freeze mode is meant to be *temporary*. As soon as we spot danger, it kicks in to protect us, then boom, off it goes and we're back to resting and digesting.

However, this isn't most people's experience; flight, flight, or freeze mode is their default, always-on setting. But staying in fear has a profound effect on the quality of our lives and our ability to be the people we deeply want and know we can be.

Think about this past week. Did you have a supersized reaction of anger, jealousy, irritability, or sadness over something small? Or maybe something big and unexpected threw you, and you were forced to make decisions, but your mind felt jumbled. You couldn't think clearly or rationally, and you just felt the spike of terror and fear.

All of these fear-based fight-or-flight responses have gotten hardwired into your system. When you have unresolved trauma, it changes how your brain works, which influences how you perceive and respond to the external world.

There are three key parts of the brain we need to look at:

- Prefrontal cortex
- Amygdala
- Limbic system

On one side of your brain, is your *prefrontal cortex*. It's associated with executive functioning skills like making decisions, thinking rationally, and problem solving. It's also connected to higher spiritual functioning and feeling like you have a purpose and meaning to your life.

Then there's the *amygdala*, which is all about fear, identifying danger, and keeping you alive.

Between these two parts of the brain is your *limbic system*, which processes memory and emotion. If your emotional state is balanced, when the amygdala signals, "Uh-oh, the sky is falling," you can take that information and still think rationally. "Okay, I know we have a problem. Here's how we'll solve it."

But for those of us with unresolved trauma, our limbic system is dysregulated, and our emotional state is unbalanced. In essence, we're locked out of the prefrontal cortex, so decision-making, rational thinking, and problem solving are gone. It's all amygdala, and when that's ruling our response it's like we're racing around, shouting, "Help! Danger! Oh my God, get away!" When we're living in this state, we have no control over our emotions, so we may often have outsized, explosive reactions to the smallest of comments or events. Out of nowhere we can be filled with rage or impatience, or we may feel a constant anxiety or depression that hums in the background of our everyday lives.

When we live with our nervous system constantly in the parasympathetic "on" fear state, we become conditioned to it. We mistakenly believe it's the right way to be. It's not, but we don't know any better. A healthier state of feeling relaxed, calm, rational, in control of our emotions, and being able to accurately assess what or who is dangerous feels wrong and uncomfortable.

In turn, we live in unhealthy, harmful states, racking up more traumas, and potentially harming other people in the process, as we're constantly being triggered. Supersized reactions to relatively minor experiences are signs that we're reacting from history.

This happened to Taylor. She was walking with her 12-year-old daughter, and Taylor was sharing what she thought was valuable advice to her kid. Her kid disagreed and did what many preadolescent kids do—she rolled her eyes at her mom. "Of course, I know that a child rolling their eyes at you is a way for them to look over you in order to find their own beliefs and ideas. It's very appropriate for a preadolescent person to be doing that," Taylor shared with us.[4]

"When my daughter rolled her eyes at me when I was sharing something important, a rage came up in me. This monster came out of me that was much bigger than what was appropriate in that moment with my child."[5]

Taylor is an early childhood family mental health specialist who focuses on trauma, so she had more tools to use than most of us and could quickly recognize how off the charts her response was. Later, Taylor worked to uncover what had happened. What she found was a memory.

Taylor grew up the youngest of five kids and raised by a single mom. She felt her voice wasn't heard as much as a kid. When her daughter rolled her eyes, it triggered the trauma of never feeling safe enough to express herself as a child. It was a "Little t" trauma that was pervasive, and she realized that unless she did more work to heal that part of her, she would risk passing trauma on to her child.

To help heal, Taylor made sure she was in situations with other adults where she could experience being heard and valued, while also mourning the child in her who never received what she needed.

It doesn't matter the exact trauma—any hidden memory and experience can arise unexpectedly. Scott, who worked in marketing for a food and beverage company, had what he considered, a normal day. He came home around 6:30 P.M., and his wife, Debbie, got home a half an hour later. He had texted her earlier and asked if she could pick up breadcrumbs on her way home. Scott was going to make spaghetti and meatballs. "Sure" came her reply.

But when Debbie got home, she walked in without the breadcrumbs. Her afternoon had gotten so busy with meetings and an unexpected office visit from her boss that she completely spaced on the grocery store. In the scheme of life, it wasn't a big deal, but it triggered an eruption in Scott. He started screaming about how he can't rely or depend on her and that he had to do everything himself. His reaction was so explosive that Debbie refused to engage with him until he cooled off.

It wasn't the first time Scott had lashed out at his wife, but it was the moment he realized he needed help in dealing with his past. When Scott was 14 years old, he lost his 8-year-old sister to cancer. It was a very sudden death. She hadn't been feeling well, so she went to the doctor. A week later she was diagnosed with an aggressive and untreatable form of cancer, and three weeks after that she was gone. Her death tore his family apart. His mom became severely depressed; his dad turned to alcohol. And Scott was left to try to take care of himself, his parents, and his 13-year-old sister.

Scott would go on to seek help from healers and therapists who worked with him slowly to unwind the painful knots inside. As he did the work and stuck with it, the explosiveness and anger began fading.

What happened to Taylor and Scott happens to so many of us. Beneath the surface, our unresolved traumas remain. The amygdala, knowing no better, keeps filtering and sorting, processing and identifying threats after threats, all connected to the past, and unless we move forward to heal, we risk being triggered.

There are moments in our lives when the amygdala is absolutely beneficial and there are experiences in this world that should trigger fear. *And* the world is filled with beauty and grace, and people and places that are safe. We need to retrain our minds and bodies to accurately discern the difference.

Your Brain Holds On to Trauma for a Reason

Have you ever wondered why you can't let go of your traumas? Most people want to. It's exhausting and painful living with trauma, and most of us would trade anything to have it disappear.

But there's a reason your mind is holding on to the trauma. "We are incredible beings, and if the brain is holding on to it, it is because it wants to," explained Brandy Gillmore, a mind and body and energy expert.[6] "When we start addressing why the brain is holding on to it now, that's when we can wholeheartedly release it."[7]

It's hard to believe that our minds want the trauma, but if we can pull back and see this as an observer, it starts to make sense. Let's look at why.

Protection

Our minds want to keep us safe. They never want us to experience that horrible event again, and so some people will hold on to trauma because remembering it—even subconsciously—keeps them safe. This is all fear driven, and as we know, fear isn't rational or logical. It's pure survival.

Energetic Coding

As Mary Morrissey, M.S., a life coach in counseling psychology, explained, every thought has a vibration that moves through the body. It goes around the brain, up and down the spinal cord, and moves into and through all the fibers, tissues, bones, and organs in your body. "When you think about the trauma, or you're afraid it could happen again, there's a vibration that gets sent throughout your body that starts getting wired and fired into your nervous system. That vibration can be so repetitive that you're feeling it when nothing happens."[8]

"The mind knows no difference between something real happening and something you're vividly imagining. There's a saying, 'where energy goes, energy flows,' so if I send my energy to rethink about this trauma, there's going to be a traumatic response in my body, which then gets hardwired into me."

As Mary explained, when this happens, your trauma gets coded into your system and your mind doesn't know how to let it go, because it's so used to living with it. Life with trauma becomes "normal" to your mind.

Stories and Beliefs

After a traumatic experience, our minds can create a story with beliefs about the world, people, and ourselves. It's meant to protect us from experiencing the trauma again. But odds are, this story has created limiting beliefs about yourself and the world around you. You may not even know these exist. We're talking beliefs like you have to be a people pleaser, you can never fail, you must sacrifice something important to you to succeed, you're undeserving of love or affection, or you must be perfect or overachieve to be accepted or respected.

We live out these stories, believing they will keep us safe from ever experiencing the original trauma again. It doesn't work. Often, we repeat similar events.

These unconscious beliefs alter how we see ourselves—and not for the better. "Imagine a child early in life hearing over and over 'you're stupid,' or 'you're useless,' or 'we're sorry we had you,' or 'you were a big mistake,'" explained Dr. Yvonne Farrell, a licensed acupuncturist and a doctor of acupuncture and Oriental medicine.[9] "These kinds of comments may not appear traumatic in the moment, but they impact our beliefs about who we are as human beings. We change our beliefs about who we are, then we're not living the lives we're meant to. We're living based on someone else's perception of who we are."[10]

As Dr. Farrell told us, this happens with "Big T" traumas too.

Addiction

Sometimes, we clearly remember our traumas and we keep the story alive by reliving it in our minds and retelling it to our friends, family members, therapists, and others. Here it's not fear it will happen again, but we get emotional hit from it. We may receive sympathy. We get a target for our anger. We get to blame someone. We get to be right. Again, we may have no awareness this is happening.

This is also a form of protection. When we shine the light on someone else, we don't have to shine it on ourselves. Meaning, we don't have to feel the pain of loneliness, hurt, rejection, betrayal, doubt, loss, or whatever we want to avoid.

It's one thing to keep going over a trauma, trying to make sense of what happened and to find the meaning from it. Processing the experience and reaching a point of "Oh, now I see, now I feel what this experience is teaching me," is a step in healing and releasing our traumas.

We get into trouble when we keep telling the same story with the same meaning. This is a sign your mind is holding on to the story for a reason. Now, if you're exploring the story to find a different perspective on what happened, then that's different. For many people on the road to recovery, this is a part of healing. They want to reclaim their stories and unwind old futile beliefs, so they can rise anew.

Trying to unearth the answers to why your mind may be holding on to trauma can be a dicey solo journey—so much of healing trauma is. That's why working with someone trained who can help you unpack the stories and work toward creating new beliefs is important.

Can't Find Trauma? Maybe It's a TBI

We've now explored the mind and body connection and what you may not realize is happening. But there's one more area to explore: traumatic brain injuries (TBIs).

TBIs are serious and can have devastating impacts. A mild case may include difficulties with speech, fatigue or drowsiness, dizziness or loss of balance, sensitivity to light or sound, or feeling depressed or anxious.[11] A moderate to severe case can include any of the symptoms of a mild one along with loss of coordination, profound confusion, slurred speech, agitation, combativeness, or other unusual behavior.[12]

When we think of a TBI, we often picture someone falling and slamming their head, being in a car accident, or getting injured playing football. It's much broader. Modern science and medicine are discovering that *any kind* of trauma below the neck can generate a group of chemicals called *cytokines* that can leak into or get transported into the brain. As Dr. Mark L. Gordon, a neuroendocrinologist who specializes in addressing the hormones of the brain and body, explained, there's a small population of these cytokines, referred to as *interleukins*, which are extremely inflammatory, and when they're produced below the neck and make it through the blood-brain barrier, they're even more inflammatory.

This inflammation interferes with other cells in the brain, spinal cord, and nervous system that can disrupt the brain chemistry and lead to personality changes, emotional disruption, mood disorders like anxiety or depression, cognitive impairment, and even PTSD. A recent study has shown that you can have inflammation in the brain *more than 17 years* after the initial injury.[13]

The implications of this are astounding. Millions of people could be walking around today—maybe even you—without having any idea they are suffering from a TBI. You may not even remember the physical trauma, since it could have been anything below your neck.

If you're struggling to trace your trauma, you may want to explore a TBI diagnosis. It's shocking how many people learn they're suffering from one when they start researching it. If you're experiencing PTSD associated with a physical trauma, you may also want to add this to the list of considerations. As Dr. Gordon explained to us, there are many people, especially veterans, who are being treated for PTSD when that's just a symptom of their brain injury. What these people need is to treat the root—the brain—and when they do, they experience remarkable turnarounds.

There are very effective treatments for TBIs. In Dr. Gordon's work, he's found that many TBI sufferers aren't producing enough estrogen, progesterone, testosterone, and growth hormone. When these hormone levels get fixed, it helps reduce the inflammation, and the brain heals. In treating civilians and active and retired military members, Dr. Gordon has found many with a TBI are low in certain minerals, including zinc, copper, and selenium, so when his patients bring these levels back up, the brain heals too.

Next, you might address inflammation from a nutritional standpoint by reducing inflammatory drinks and high-fat foods, alcohol, and sugar, and maybe (at the direction of your doctor) take supplements, such as fish oil, vitamin D, and DHA. All of this combined can act like jet fuel, and your healing will take off.

There are some remarkable stories of people who have healed their TBIs. Now, there is no "pop the red pill and all will be well" approach. It's a multifaceted healing plan that's individualized depending on what you need. There's also neurotherapy, heart rate variability training, infrared saunas, and other treatments that some people use—as a stand-alone or in combination with others.

THE ROAD TO RECOVERY

Sundar finally found relief. It came from more than one place.

A friend suggested he try craniosacral therapy, a light-touch healing modality. Sundar had always been skeptical of alternative therapies, but he was desperate. His body quickly took to it, and after a few sessions, he started to notice the constant tension and pressure in his body, neck, and head ease.

Simultaneously, he sought help from a psychotherapist who used inner-child healing and guided imagery to explore Sundar's emotions and his early life, where Sundar uncovered an intense feeling of self-criticism that had formed around a belief about how to stay safe. When Sundar was about eight years old, he did something that almost got him killed. The experience itself was terrifying and traumatic for him, but it was made more difficult because of how furious he perceived his parents were with him, though, most likely, his parents were scared. "How could you be so stupid? What were you thinking?" they had screamed.

From that experience, Sundar's mind had created a story and a belief that told him, "I can't trust myself. I could end up killing myself. I need to make sure that I'm listening and getting feedback and criticism from other people all the time."

Sundar had also struggled with belonging. His parents had moved to the United States when he was four years old. Growing up, he was often picked on and teased by the other neighborhood kids who called him a "sand n****r." They'd make fun of him because his parents didn't speak English very well, and when they were bringing PB&J sandwiches for lunch, he was bringing curries that "smelled funny" to the other kids. Sundar learned that if he wanted to be accepted, he needed to fit in—as best as he could. So he'd take the criticisms that came from teasing and use them to change his behaviors and how he showed up in the world.

These experiences had combined to create a life filled with criticism—from himself and others. The pain was too much for Sundar to hold inside, and so it came out in migraines. Sundar had to work to change the underlying beliefs from "I need criticism to stay safe and accepted" to "I can trust myself to know what I need and who I am in every breath."

Sundar's therapist had suggested he adopt self-nurturing practices, including guided meditation, spending time in nature, and positive affirmations like "I am willing to be healthy," "I am willing to experience life without migraines," and "I am willing to trust myself." He also started practicing martial arts, which boosted his confidence and self-esteem. Slowly, his self-image changed.

"I am capable of handling any experience that happens in my life," Sundar began telling himself. To help build more trust, he made lists of everything he was good at. Instead of focusing on criticisms and what he could do better, he directed his energy toward his talents, skills, and gifts, acknowledging them and himself for the first time.

It was a process, but Sundar's migraines did improve and so did his situation at the hospital. He went six months before an episode struck, but when it did, he saw it as a signal that he needed to manage his stress and practice more self-care. He had taken on extra shifts since it was the holidays.

Overall, the more Sundar focused on rewriting his stories and beliefs, and keeping his mind and body healthy and strong, the more he lived migraine-free. He figured he'd always have to work on and be vigilant with his thoughts and beliefs and health, but this didn't bother him. It felt good to take care of his mind and body and to see the positive changes.

Sundar's story teaches us that to release trauma, sometimes we have to go into our minds to understand the stories and meanings we may have unintentionally created. The mind-body connection is real and we have to work with both to heal both. That doesn't mean releasing trauma happens instantly. Like Sundar, we may need to spend multiple sessions working with a trusted ally, and we may have to try multiple treatments to give our minds and bodies the care they need to slowly let go of the stored pain. But little by little, it can happen, and we can change our lives in the process.

No matter how long you've carried your pain, you will always have the chance to let it go. Sundar teaches us that when our minds and bodies are ready, we can release the stored pain and reclaim our health and vitality.

REFLECTIONS

As you think about this chapter, tune in to your body. How does it feel? Do you have certain weak spots that flare up often? If so, what are they? Do you regularly pull or strain a muscle? If so, list them. Do you usually feel relaxed, or does it seem like you're anxious or stressed more often than not? Do you suffer from an illness that Western doctors struggle to treat? Spend a few minutes quietly considering how your body feels in the moment and historically. Keep a list of recurring aches and pains, especially any that you've had since childhood, and note if you remember any symptoms occurring after a difficult experience or event. This list may become the road map to unwinding your trauma.

SAGE WISDOM

"There's this beautiful relationship between the body and the psyche where when we're in a situation that feels too much for our psyches to bear, the body says, 'I'll take that, so you can keep going, so you can survive this.'"

—Taylor Ross

CHAPTER 3

MANIFESTING IN THE GUT

Mary, 52, was 75 pounds overweight.

Weight struggles were nothing new. Her parents put her on a diet when she was 13, and she had been going up and down the scales ever since. Some diets, she'd lose the weight, but she could never keep it off, and when the scale crept back up, it eventually landed on a higher number than before.

It was demoralizing and embarrassing.

It wasn't just the weight; it was everything that went along with it too. Mary felt so uncomfortable in her body. She was anxious all the time, so her doctor put her on an antianxiety medication. She was also deeply exhausted. She had to use sugar and caffeine to get going in the morning for her job as the chief financial officer of a college. And she had to use pills and sometimes alcohol to shut off her mind, but her nights were still restless.

Mary would sometimes feel queasy and have sharp, stabbing pains, and her bowels were never regular. She'd get intense acid reflux too. She'd seen a gastrointestinal specialist who diagnosed her with irritable bowel syndrome.

Five years before, Mary had gotten divorced, and she really wanted to start dating again, but she was haunted by the thought, *Who would want to date me like this?* She knew she didn't want to go on living with all of these health challenges, but she had no idea where or how to start addressing them. And a part of her wondered, *Is change even possible, or is it too late?*

OUR TRIALS

Constipation, diarrhea, and other "untreatable" stomach pains often get shrugged off. If we go to see a Western doctor, they may diagnosis you with irritable bowel syndrome (IBS), which doesn't have a cure. For most of our stomach issues, we tell ourselves, "it's a part of life."

Except it's not.

Odd stomach and bowel ailments can be symptoms of trauma that have manifested as gastrointestinal issues and inflammation. In the last decade, researchers have uncovered a connection between trauma, chronic stress, and the gut. Research from the Mayo Clinic has found childhood and adult traumas were more common among IBS sufferers.[1] We're also beginning to learn about the links between unresolved trauma and autoimmune diseases, and trauma and emotional eating (including binge eating and overeating), or struggles losing weight.

Gut issues, autoimmune diseases, and weight-loss problems are real, and your unresolved traumas may be the cause. Whatever happens, keep searching for answers. Don't let any medical professional tell you to "just live with it" or "sorry, there's nothing we can do." Don't believe that for a second. You deserve to live symptom free. You deserve to have a functioning and healthy gut and immune system. You deserve to experience life at a weight that is healthy and right for your body.

Like so many issues, fixing your gut and what trauma has done to it may take more than one day. That's normal. Besides, the most rewarding experiences in life take time. Stories of instant weight loss, get rich quick, and overnight sensations are myths. In this chapter, we're going to walk you through what may be happening in your gut and the potential links to trauma so you can better understand the inner workings of your body.

Ultimately, it requires you to slow down and listen to what your gut is telling you. Pay attention to whether you're often bloated, constipated, or have diarrhea. Don't just shrug off these gastrointestinal issues. Don't just throw up your hands with autoimmune diseases or weight-loss struggles.

Take the time you need to understand and hear what your gut is telling you. By slowing down, listening, and noticing, you'll hear the wisdom of your body.

THE AWAKENINGS

Your Gut May Be Inflamed

The story of your gut begins with your microbiome, which consists of hundreds of good and bad bacteria, viruses, fungi, and other tiny microbes that live in your stomach, colon, and entire gastrointestinal tract. It helps you to digest your food into minerals, vitamins, and nutrients that your body needs. A healthy microbiome has all of these tiny organisms living in balance and harmony. An unhealthy microbiome is one that's out of balance.

There are a number of possible causes for imbalance, including diet. If you eat a lot of sugary, processed, high-fat foods, then your bad bacteria will love you. Toxins can also disrupt the balance, and so can stress.

The more you live in the fight, flight, or freeze zone, the more you risk disrupting your microbiome and creating an environment where inflammation skyrockets. Inflammation is a natural part of your body's defense mechanism. It's an immune response that's created when there's a physical injury. It's also created when an intruder or threat is identified. When something doesn't belong in our bodies—a virus, bacteria, toxin, or processed food—our immune system fires off cells, including those cytokines we previously mentioned, to seek and destroy.

We need to have both an immune response and inflammation. But having too much of it can cause physical symptoms such as irritable bowel syndrome, constipation, nausea, diarrhea, and pain.

When your microbiome is off, it can also create problems in other parts of your body such as your brain. Your gut and brain are connected through the *polyvagal pathway*, which is a nerve pathway.

Prolonged stress and living in fight, flight, or freeze will produce a lot of cortisol. This cortisol can affect the gut lining. Think of your gut lining as a barrier that regulates what leaves your gut and gets into the blood stream to be carried to other organs. In a healthy micro-biome, that gut lining is solid. Nothing gets through that shouldn't.

An unhealthy microbiome mixed with increases of cortisol can weaken the gut lining and eventually lead to *leaky gut*, where bacteria, particles, undigested food molecules, fungi, and other elements can leak from the gut into the bloodstream and get carried throughout the body where they shouldn't be. Because of the direct link between the gut and brain, all the things that should stay in the gut travel through the polyvagal pathway and hit the brain, leading to exhaustion, brain fog, confusion, and depression.

Remember your immune system. When it picks up a threat, it's going to mount a defense. When it notices that bad bacteria have leaked out of the gut, it's going to send its warriors to fight off the invader, and that creates more inflammation. Now you have inflammation spreading from your gut through your body.

If this sounds exhausting, it is, and we're not done. When you're living in stress all the time and that cortisol is pumping, it affects your gut's ability to produce *serotonin*, the happy chemical. We often associate serotonin with the brain, but the chemical is actually produced in your gut. Not only does your gut feel funky because of all of this inflammation, now you feel sad and depressed too. The impacts of trauma truly reverberate in unpredictable yet very costly ways.

We admit, this can seem very complicated and messy; however, there is a solution. People suffering from chronic digestive and stomach problems have seen very positive results when they clean up their microbiome. You can do a lot of this on your own too.

First, you can help to rebalance your microbiome through diet. Switching to anti-inflammatory foods such as berries (strawberries, raspberries, blueberries, blackberries), fatty fish (salmon, mackerel, sardines), broccoli, avocados, and green tea can help. As you increase your intake of anti-inflammatory foods, eliminate the ones that can often cause reactions, including dairy, eggs, refined carbohydrates, gluten, vegetable and seed oils, and sugar. Second, you can add more pre- and probiotics to your diet. These two steps alone can help you to balance your microbiome.

If you want to take it further, you can also seek out a functional medicine practitioner who may be able to help measure your vitamin, mineral, and nutrient levels, and to check for any bacteria or fungal imbalances.

These steps may also help clear up any brain fog, mood changes, headaches, and other cognitive functions that could be caused by an unhappy gut.

Then when you add resolving your underlying traumas to this mix, you can create an even more powerful effect that can dramatically change how you feel and move through this world.

Trauma, Inflammation, and the Potential Connection to Autoimmune Diseases

When a therapist friend sent the ACE Study to Dr. Jorina Elbers, a pediatric neurologist, she was blown away. "I saw the title of the study about adverse childhood experiences and read the abstract and thought, 'Wow, this is amazing! This is finally coming forward.' I searched to see what journal this was published in and when, and I was shocked. It was over 20 years ago, and I thought, 'How did this not get traction?'"[2]

The ACE Study, conducted between 1995 and 1997, was a landmark study by the Center for Disease Control and Prevention and Kaiser Permanente's Health Appraisal Clinic that surveyed 17,000 adults. The study looked at the negative effect that adverse childhood experiences could have on our health as we got older. It identified 10 experiences and asked participants to note how many they had been exposed to before the age of 18.

The experiences included:

- Physical, sexual, and emotional abuse
- Physical or emotional neglect
- Losing a parent such as through divorce
- Being exposed to domestic violence between your parents
- Having a parent with a mental illness like depression
- Having a member of the household who abuses substances such as alcohol or drugs
- Having a member of the household in jail

The study found that 64 percent of the participants had at least one adverse childhood experience.[3] It also found that people with a high ACE score (one point for each experience) may be at a higher risk for developing autoimmune diseases.[4] More studies have since connected the same dots. Research has found that people suffering from PTSD are also at a higher risk for autoimmune diseases.[5]

Is there a direct correlation between your autoimmune disease and your trauma? Not necessarily. Your trauma may not cause the disease, but it could play a factor. Medical science is still understanding the intimate connection between the microbiome, inflammation, and the immune system. About 60–70 percent of your immune system is located in the gut.[6]

But it's not just these adverse childhood traumas that place people at risk—chronic stress from any and all traumas does too.[7] Chronic stress, as we noted, can increase the inflammation in your body. Inflammation has been found to play a role in autoimmune diseases.[8]

If you're suffering from Lyme disease, rheumatoid arthritis, multiple sclerosis, or one of the other 70–80 autoimmune diseases, you may want to consider your trauma history. "I work a lot with people with autoimmune disease, and there are three Ps for everyone with autoimmunity: perfectionism, people pleasing, and the poison of holding on to past pain," explained Dr. Keesha Ewers, the founder of the Academy for Integrative Medicine, an integrative medicine expert, doctor of sexology, trauma-informed psychotherapist, and board-certified functional medicine provider.[9]

Autoimmune diseases can seem like a beast to deal with, precisely because most Western medical doctors don't have a clue how to treat them. Understanding our traumas and learning how to heal them could be the secret to unlocking many of our autoimmune issues.

Your Vagus Nerve May Have Shut Down

When we talk about living in a constant state of stress, most people get it—and many feel there's nothing they can do about it.

If it feels impossible to switch your nervous system, that's because it may actually be impossible.

The vagus nerve, also known as the "wanderer nerve," runs from the brainstem through the neck and thorax, and into the stomach.[10] It carries messages from the gut, liver, heart, and lungs to the brain, and it's responsible for organ functions such as digestion and heartbeat.[11]

The vagus nerve is the main contributor to your parasympathetic nervous system. It's responsible for monitoring your prefrontal cortex, the amygdala, and the limbic system for threats. When it's clear and safe, the vagus nerve reports the information to the nervous system and you shift into parasympathetic rest-and-digest mode.[12]

The challenge we're facing with unresolved trauma is that our vagus nerve has shut down. It's closed for business, so we can't shift into rest and digest. "The vagus nerve is the single most important nerve in the body that keeps our system healthy and regulated," explained Dr. Jorina Elbers. "People think that the sympathetic nervous system is the problem. In fact, the first thing that happens within milliseconds of a threat response in the amygdala is the vagus nerve, which drops out. The activity of this nerve, which is trying to keep us healthy, is not online to keep the system in check. Then the sympathetic nervous system takes over and keeps us in fight or flight."

What Dr. Elbers is describing is also known as the *polyvagal theory*, as put forward by Stephen Porges, a professor of psychiatry. The theory focuses on the freeze and immobilize response in our nervous system, which Porges says is a very common reaction for trauma survivors. It's not about the trauma itself, but our reaction to it.

When the vagus nerve goes silent, it's very difficult for us to shift into digest and rest, so we stay in fight, flight, or freeze. But according to Dr. Elbers and other experts, there are a number of treatments aimed at bringing the vagus nerve back to life. Cognitive thought therapy, dialectical behavior therapy, eye movement desensitization reprocessing, somatic experiencing, narrative or exposure work, breath worth, and heart math, which uses heart rate variability and biofeedback to teach emotional regulation and reconnect to a positive emotion, are just some of the tools out there.

Your Digestion May Be Dysregulated

According to the Centers for Disease Control, over 70 percent of Americans over the age of 20 are overweight or obese.[13] That's a shocking figure when you think about how much we know about healthy lifestyles, exercise, and eating clean, wholesome, and nutritious food.

When we saw that number, we wondered: How many people are suffering from trauma? How many people aren't struggling with weight but trauma issues?

As a society, we talk about extra weight as if it's the problem, but what if it was just a sign pointing to the real underlying issue? And what if unresolved trauma changes the body's chemistry in very real and profound ways?

Human beings may have evolved significantly since our hunter-gatherer days, but our systems remain primitive. Anytime you eat, your system is asking this basic question: "Do I feel safe enough to rest and digest?" It's a yes or no response. That's it.

When your nervous system gets stuck operating in its stress mode, then you get a lot of cortisol. Too much of it can signal to your body that it needs to store weight. That's because your survival response has kicked in. This is ancient ancestor stuff. If there was a famine, drought, or the hunting and gathering was poor, a stress response would get triggered. "No food? We'd better slow down our metabolism, stop digesting food or building muscle, and store fat to survive."

Too much cortisol also blunts the body's ability to register pleasure. That was a good thing for our ancestors. If they were being chased by a bear, they didn't want to get sidetracked by a plump strawberry patch. Flash forward to today. You come home from work and it was rough. What do you do? You reach for something to eat. Food will make you feel better—there's a reason why we call some dishes "comfort food."

But if you're stressed and your body's pumping cortisol, you won't feel comforted by that food, because you can't. You don't realize this, so you reach for an extra serving, maybe two. You're driven to eat more because your brain is driving you. "If the brain's not getting the pleasure it seeks, it keeps going after it," said Marc David, founder of the Institute for the Psychology of Eating, who specializes in eating psychology and how to work with weight, body image, binge eating, and emotional eating.[14] "But then I say to myself, 'I'm a willpower weakling. There's something wrong with me. I can't stop myself. I have a problem.' No, your appetite is fine. What's happening is you're under stress."[15]

We'll add one more hormone to this recipe, and that's insulin. Insulin arrives when you eat and delivers the glucose (sugar) from your food to the millions of cells, which use it as fuel to energize your body. If you overeat, at some point your cells will be maxed out. They won't need more energy, but there's still a ton of glucose floating around, and your insulin has to do something with it—cut to converting and storing it as fat.

There's a science of the body that's at play, preventing you from losing extra weight. As long as you remain trapped in the fear-based fight, flight, or freeze zone, you will struggle to get into the rest-and-digest state, and you will continue to grapple with these extra pounds.

The excess pounds aren't about shame or guilt or self-blame. *You* haven't done anything wrong. It's the trauma that has you off center and your digestion dysregulated.

This isn't about healing your weight; it's about healing your trauma. Making the connection between your weight struggles and your trauma is a powerful healing force by itself. When we understand and accept that our body is normal and it's operating the way it's been programmed, it creates understanding, compassion, and more empathy.

Of course, it's important to eat healthy, wholesome foods (preferably organic) and to move your body. These are two foundational pillars of healthy living and strengthening our resiliency, so we have the capacity to cope and thrive no matter what experiences we encounter.

Your Extra Weight Could Be Protecting You

When we think about our gut, we think food. When we think food, we often think of weight, which is one of the most difficult health topics to talk about and figure out.

In our last book, *Exhausted*, we talked about how our bodies use fat to store toxins so they don't poison us. In our *Exhausted* story, our body fat was actually the hero and heroine of our lives.

Well, sit tight, because in our trauma story, your body fat plays the same starring role, even if the medical community is still playing catch-up to this idea. As Marc David explained, "If you have a headache, there's probably a thousand reasons why. It could be stress-related, it could be food-related, it could be allergies, it could be you have a brain tumor. When it comes to weight, science is still in the dark ages. And when we think of extra weight, medical science goes: calories in, calories out, eat less, exercise more, and if you do that, you're going to lose weight. We have been getting that wisdom since the 1960s, and it doesn't work."

People try to lose weight. They eat less or go on some fad diet, exercise like a fiend, and maybe they shed the weight, but when they check in a year later, they're back where they started—possibly with more weight on the scale. When your weight-loss plan doesn't work, how do you feel? Do you feel ashamed, like there's something wrong with you, you're weak, or you lack the willpower and discipline?

Do you stare in the mirror, pointing the finger at yourself, believing you're broken?

From here, it's a downward spiral. You feel ashamed of yourself because of the extra weight and start hating yourself because you can't fix what science and medicine says you should be able to fix.

If you've struggled mightily for years, decades even, with weight issues, know this: there is nothing wrong with you or your body. Your body is actually doing something beautiful—it's protecting you from the pain, from the toxins that are stored within whatever traumas you've experienced.

Traumas are undigested experiences.

Any trauma, experienced at any moment in your life, can trigger your body to store it as fat.

"When we have chronic day in, day out stress, one of the ways that the body or the brain perceives that is, 'I'm going to survive longer if I'm bigger,'" Marc David said.[16] "Nature knows that the bigger the creature you are, the more fearsome you are. Look at any animals fighting. Look at your dog. What's the first thing that happens? Their hair stands up. The dog starts to grow. You want to look big. The bigger the creature, the better chance you have of survival. Unbeknownst to the unconscious mind in a long-term stress response, a bigger body equals 'I am safe.'"[17]

Unconsciously, our bodies hold on to extra weight as a defensive, protective measure against future threats. If you were a young man, woman, or small child, or if you were sexually or physically abused or the threat was there, then your subconscious created a story and belief that "if I'm bigger, I'm less of a target." For women, subconsciously they may also be absorbing societal cues that say "men find slender, thin women sexually attractive." If you carry extra weight, then it may be ingrained in you to think that you are less likely to be abused again.

Holding on to weight is a survival strategy. It's the wisdom of your body keeping you safe and protecting you.

We know this may be a big ask right now, but try to see your weight through a different lens. It isn't the enemy; it's been an ally doing everything it can to keep you safe until the moment when you're ready to lay down your shield.

Maybe, just maybe, *this* is the beginning of doing just that.

THE ROAD TO RECOVERY

Mary wasn't ready to give up, so she saw a functional medicine practitioner who tested her for everything—hormonal imbalance, food sensitivities, adrenals, and mold sensitivities, and to see if her microbiome was unbalanced with any fungi, bacteria, or virus that was causing the harm.

All the tests came back normal.

That's when her doctor asked about any past traumas.

At the age of 12, Mary's uncle began molesting her. He told her he'd kill her if she told anyone. With no outlet and no idea how to process the experience, Mary turned to food. The 12-year-old voice that was still inside had kept telling her, "Just eat. You'll feel better," even though she really didn't, but for a moment she would.

Mary's doctor suggested she do a deep-dive, intensive one-week small group retreat, followed by regular check-ins and visits and EMDR sessions. During that first week, Mary worked to unpack some of the reasons around why she ate. She realized she never, *ever* wanted to be beautiful or sexy or attractive because she judged that her beauty had gotten her molested.

On one of the last days, Mary's doctor led the group in a guided meditation. In her meditation, Mary took herself to a pier on a marina, and she looked at herself and said, "I'm really beautiful. My weight really got me to this point where I could come here."

"What are you seeing?" Mary's doctor asked.

"I looked at the dark next to me, and it's me, and I'm thin, and I'm beautiful, and she's inviting me to come over."

When Mary opened her eyes she said, "I feel clean, because I don't feel dirty."

After the one-week intensive, Mary also began eye movement desensitization reprogramming (EMDR), and she adopted an anti-inflammation diet, cutting back on coffee and cutting out sugar. Within six weeks, Mary had lost 15 pounds, she was sleeping more, and she felt lighter, happier, and had self-love and appreciation that was wholly new to her.

Mary stuck with her treatments and eventually moved to a maintenance plan with her doctor. She still had trauma triggers, so her road to recovery wasn't a straight shot (let's be real: it never is), but she learned how to identify them and how to practice self-care. Over the next couple of years, Mary's weight continued to fall, and she kept it off as she learned that she no longer needed it to protect a wound.

Trauma can hide in our bodies in many ways. Mary's story shows us that sometimes it's in the extra pounds we carry and our relationship to food. Undigested traumatic experiences can manifest themselves in harmful physical ailments, excess weight, and autoimmune diseases. Her story also teaches us that when we take small steps to unwind the traumas and integrate them, then the physical pain will likely subside too. This is the complete mind-body transformation, and it happens when we turn, face the trauma, and take steps to work our way through them.

REFLECTIONS

Gut issues can be a sign of stored trauma manifested as physical conditions, so consider if you suffer from strange, inexplicable gut issues that seem immune to treatments. Do you have an autoimmune disease? Do you struggle with weight issues? Spend a few minutes quietly focused inward and listen to what your gut may be trying to tell you. Reflect on how you responded to this chapter too. If you found yourself pausing or thinking *that's interesting* or *that sounds like me*, jot that down. Your gut health can give you powerful clues to help you see and eventually release your trauma—you just have to quiet your mind to hear the messages.

SAGE WISDOM

"Trauma disconnects us from ourselves and our life force. We disconnect out of survival. We don't want to feel the pain. But when we shut down the painful part of ourselves, we also shut down the joyous part, the liveliness in us. We need to go beyond our traumas to feel our life force again, to be in touch with that sense of awe and joy for being alive."

—Dr. Joanne Barron

CHAPTER 4

BIRTH, CHILDHOOD, AND PARENTING

Michael had plateaued.

For six months, he had been working with a functional medicine practitioner to help address his chronic stress, fatigue, and out-of-control temper. When he first went to the doctor's, he felt like he was barely holding his life together. In his mid-40s, he was juggling being a partner at his law firm, a husband, and a father to four kids between the ages of 2 and 10.

With his doctor's help and under her guidance, he was taking supplements to address mineral deficiencies. He had reduced his work hours, setting aside family-only time every day. He was sleeping better, going to bed earlier, and getting up later. He had stopped training for a marathon and had switched to cycling during his lunch break and hikes on the weekend with the family.

He felt like he was about 75 percent of the way back to optimal health. But he couldn't shake the tension and impatience. He still snapped and would lose his temper at little things. He knew he was overreacting, but he couldn't control it.

He needed something more to get him the rest of the way there, but he had no idea what that was.

OUR TRIALS

World, we have a problem, and it's childhood trauma.

It is truly shocking—and heartbreaking—to think of how many of us have experienced trauma, and how it keeps getting passed down from generation to generation. No one gets out of childhood without *some* traumatic experiences. Even if you think you had the greatest parents or parent ever and that you were raised in a stable, loving environment, you likely still walked out of your early years with something that's wedged itself in your mind and body.

Just think back to your school years. What was the playground like? What was the bus ride or walk to school like? What was it like during gym? What about after school? Did you ever get picked last for kickball, or not make the baseball team or school play? Were you ever picked on? Did you ever want to sit next to someone or be friends, and they rejected you? Ever feel betrayed by a friend? Ever feel misunderstood by your parents or not listened to? Ever wish your mom or dad were around more? Did a friend, parent, or loved one die or get really sick? Were you in an accident?

We could fill this chapter with *so many* experiences that could have left you scarred—the "Big T" and "Little t" ones. "Little t" traumas can be especially tough, because we may not even recognize them—that's how common and frequent they could have been. When we're exposed to an event or message repeatedly, we become desensitized. Feeling rejected, abandoned, betrayed, teased, stupid, lazy, ugly, hurt—it just becomes how life is.

We leave so much in our pasts, for good reason, but we're also leaving many unresolved and unhealed traumas that absolutely need to be brought into the light if we have any hope of living to our highest potential.

When we roll into adulthood with all our unresolved traumas, it makes coping with life so much harder for us. In our modern world, we're inundated 24/7 with outrageous expectations. We live in an always-on, always-be-hustling, never-slow-down mode. We've got kids, marriages, relationships, careers, mortgages, rents, grandchildren, aging parents, car loans, student loans—the list keeps growing while our capacity to deal shrinks.

From birth to childhood to adulthood, eventually it becomes too much for our systems. Imagine a glass continually being filled with water. If you don't find a way to release some of it, eventually it will spill over.

We sincerely believe everyone has a purpose in this world, and everyone is meant to reach their full potential—to be creative, caring, and compassionate, and to learn, grow, and evolve—on this journey of being human. But we can't do it if we don't deal with our childhood scars. For all the moms and dads out there, if you don't heal these wounds, you could also repeat and pass them on to your kiddos—and we know, you don't want to do that.

This chapter is about *clarity*. It's about accepting that there were likely childhood experiences that your little self couldn't process, but that your big self can. In this chapter, we're going to help light your path back to the original injury. We're going to highlight some of the less-talked-about experiences in the preverbal years, unintentional trauma from well-meaning parents and caregivers, and how our little selves probably created powerful stories and beliefs about our experiences that we have carried into our adult years.

For some of us, our childhood traumas are easily and quickly spotted. For others, not so much, and often we need to go back with the help and guidance of a trusted healer who creates a safe space for us. If you read this chapter and you're stumped about the early years, or if you work with a healer and you can't find a memory, that's okay. There may not be a specific memory, event, or even a chain of them that you ever recall.

And if going back into your past is too traumatic or retriggering, that's okay too. If you need to skip this chapter, go for it. You may need to double-back to it later down the road—that's okay too. The most important thing you can do is take care of yourself.

Your path is *your* path. There is no set time frame for your journey, so never force yourself to do something when it's not time or it doesn't feel right.

THE AWAKENINGS

You Can Experience Trauma Before You Can Remember

Trauma can get coded into our systems long before our conscious memories kick in. We're going to look at four major moments in your early history that the experts we spoke to said can have an outsized impact on the trajectory of your life.

Conception and Pregnancy

We are energy, so it's worth thinking about the energy surrounding your parents when you were conceived. Were they happy and content and filled with love, using sex as the ultimate act in intimacy and connection? Or were they angry, upset, or anxious, using sex as a distraction from their pain? (Granted, most of us will not feel comfortable asking our parents, "Hey, were you and Mom/Dad in sync when you made me?" but if you can find out what life was like for them before you arrived on the scene, that can be great knowledge.)

Research has found that when we're in the womb, our mothers' mental and emotional states and their environments can affect how we develop after we're born.[1] What was your mom's pregnancy like? Was Mom relaxed, peaceful, and filled with love while she carried you, or was she anxious, pushed to the brink of exhaustion? What was Mom's relationship like with her partner? Was it healthy and supportive, or was it abusive and fear-ridden?

Part of this story has to do with what information our mothers pass to us while they're carrying us, including telling our immune systems what to react to and what foods are safe to eat. Our mothers aren't conscious of this; it's biologically driven so that we have the best chance to survive.

The more our mothers experienced a state of well-being—physiological, psychological, emotional—the more capacity we had to recognize and mimic that on the outside. The reverse is true too. The more we experienced fear and anxiety, the more predisposed we became to these states once we came into the world.

During Birth

For some babies, their entrance into the world was traumatic. "If the mother is anxious, depressed, if she's frightened for her life, the infant in uterus is feeling that, they're getting all of that transferred to them at a cellular level during the birth process," explained Dr. Joanne Barron, a licensed clinical psychologist.[2]

Sometimes birth doesn't go smoothly. For instance, babies who are born with their umbilical cords wrapped around their necks come into the world choking, gasping for air, frightened for their lives. As an adult, you won't remember this, but your body will remember this terrorizing introduction into this world.

As a result, you may spend your entire life experiencing a profound anxiety and having no idea where it came from. You may feel disconnected from your body, emotions, and people in your life because you don't know what it feels like to be relaxed and to feel safe. This can trace back to your first experience in this new world.

Some of the experts we spoke with mentioned other experiences at birth that could potentially affect people in similar ways like C-sections or being born prematurely and having to stay in a neonatal care unit. Sometimes the act of being born before being ready can leave a trauma imprint. Babies born premature may not have been able to have been held or had the close touch and comfort of their mother or primary caregiver when they needed it.

Being touched, held, spoken to softly, or gazed at with love is how a baby knows it's safe, and that sensation—that energy—gets absorbed by them. When they don't immediately receive that, they miss out on learning that the world is safe for them and that they are loved, cared, and secure. While it may have been unavoidable and no one's fault, if that was your entry into this realm, you may still carry the underlying feeling that the world is a frightening place and you're all alone in it.

Early Weeks after Birth

Experts have found that the best practices for healthy humans is for the baby to have quiet downtime in the early weeks after birth with their mother and other caregivers. This is a bonding period, where skin-to-skin contact, eye gazing, making little sounds back and forth, and just being with each other form healthy attachments.

Yet, for so many of us, the early formative bonding experience wasn't there, so we didn't absorb how to attach in a healthy and secure way to our primary caregiver. This was devastating for our little systems, which coded it as "I don't get the support I need."

Many adults today would wager that they grew up in environments like this—and that kids are still being raised in them. As a society, we've failed. We've "blown off" how important this early phase of bonding and caregiving is. This is when the foundation for our lives going forward gets set. We either know what it's like to bond deeply with our mothers and primary caregivers, knowing that we're safe and loved and secured—or we don't. We will carry whatever we're given here with us going forward.

If we miss the bonding here, then later, as we grow, our systems won't learn how to create healthy attachments with others, resulting in insecurity and feeling unsupported in life. As adults, we have to go in and rewire the hardwire. It's not impossible. You can learn to do it, but it's challenging and it takes constant practice.

Up to 12 months

When an infant is hungry, cold, tired, or just plain uncomfortable in their body, they cry. That's how they let their mother or primary caregiver know that they need something. If that need goes unmet, they wail. They're experiencing a difficult, stressful moment, and their primary caregiver has gone MIA or can't figure out what they need.

The longer this goes on, the more the infant moves into a heightened distressed state, and the more upset they become. Their tiny nervous system is sending out fear, rage, and separation distress signals. If their needs still go unmet, at some point, the fear and distress become too much to tolerate. Cue the vagus nerve, which comes online and flips the failsafe switch, disconnecting the infant from their body and emotions and immobilizing them.

Now it's up to the primary caregiver to step in and repair the circuits. They've got to pick up the baby, soothe them, hold them, reconnect with them, calm them down, and slowly bring them back into their body and emotions. Here, the primary caregiver is teaching the baby's nervous system how to self-soothe. The same thing happens with small children too.

This act between the primary caregiver and the infant is so important because during the first year after a baby is born, the nervous system is still developing. They don't know how to self-soothe; they learn it from their primary caregiver, who teaches the baby how to feel safe in the world and their bodies. Babies get that sense of safety and well-being and peace when they're being held, spoken to in a calm, soothing tone, and engaged with their primary caregiver who provides what they need.

Babies also use their primary caregiver's nervous system to calm down. In a perfect world, the primary caregiver's nervous system will be relaxed, calm, and peaceful, so the baby can mirror that state too.

We would have learned how to self-soothe, calm our nervous systems, and feel safe in our bodies and the world from our primary caregiver.

But if they were a no-show or were constantly chaotic, stressed, strung out, angry, or frustrated, even if unavoidable or by no fault of their own, then our nervous system would not have been taught what peaceful, restful, and relaxed feels like. This would have been hugely traumatic to our systems.

❖

If you're wondering, *How am I supposed to know if any of these things happened?* No worries, you don't have to remember. Most people don't. If you feel comfortable, you can ask family members what they remember. Maybe someone recalls if you were difficult to soothe or that life at home with your parents or caregiver was stressful.

If you don't have stories or feel uncomfortable asking for them, again, no big deal. Ask yourself if you can remember feeling relaxed and peaceful as a kid. If you think back, and you can hardly ever remember feeling chill and if you're like "I've always been like this," then these could be signs that your nervous system didn't get the training it needed in those very early stages.

Seeking a trained therapist who you can feel safe with and who can teach you techniques to move your nervous system into a relaxed state can be hugely beneficial. Mindfulness, meditation, yoga, and qi-gong practices can also teach your system how to unwind and relax. These tools rewire, retrain, and redevelop your inner system to know love, security, safety, and eventually healthy relationships and bonds with other people.

When you miss out on key experiences with your parents or primary caregivers, it is painful. In some ways, pain, discomfort, insecurity, isolation, and disconnection are all you may have ever known or experienced. But the beauty of life is that it's never too late to learn. You can retrain and reteach yourself how to feel secure, protected, safe, loved, connected, and comfortable in this world, with yourself, and with other people.

We can regenerate our lives and chart a new future for ourselves. Sure, it can take work—a lot of it—but if you believe there's a better way and a chance for a different path, then you will find it.

You May Have Unintentional Trauma from Your Parents

There are some truly horrible parents in this world who have done horrendous acts and treated their kids in horrifying ways. These parents can and often do leave deep wounds that take a lot of work to heal. If you were raised by one of these people, you know it.

But then there are parents who don't fit the stereotypical "bad parent" role, yet their parenting styles can unintentionally leave trauma scars that are very difficult to spot—because you don't think of your mom or dad that way. You think of them as "good people." They were generally loving, and they wanted the best for you. They probably tried their hardest to give you a good life, most likely a better one than what they had experienced growing up.

Yet, life still happened, and they may have fallen short in ways they never intended or expected. Maybe they carried their own traumas, had more stress than they could handle, or lacked the resiliency to manage what life threw at them.

For whatever reason, maybe your caregivers weren't able to give you what you needed or in the way you needed it.

Dave Richo, a psychotherapist, says that everyone comes into the world seeking "The Five Basic Needs" from their caregivers. That includes:

1. **Attention.** We enter the world without a vocabulary. Crying was the only way to make our needs known, and we had to have caregivers who could understand us. This meant they had to pay attention to us. By doing so, they should—theoretically—have learned when we needed to be fed, be held, or have our diapers changed.

2. **Affection.** Our brains are not fully developed in the womb. Physical affection, cuddling, and being held by our caregivers helps our brains to develop.

3. **Appreciation.** We need to have a sense that we are valuable, that our lives are valuable just because we are human. This gives us a sense of safety and security. We know that we won't be thrown away or rejected.

4. **Acceptance.** As we went from babies to toddlers to little kids, our personalities began emerging, and we needed our caregivers to accept us just as we were and not try to change or mold us into who they thought we should be. We needed to be met with curiosity, with our caregivers wanting to get to know who we were and then welcoming us.

5. **Allowing.** This relates to the beginning of our independence. At first, we depended on our caregivers for everything, but then we learned to crawl, then walk, then we went to school, and then eventually, flash forward many years, we moved out. This is the journey most of us make. We needed our caregivers to have welcomed and encouraged these transitions to interdependence instead of keeping us dependent by clinging to us.[3]

According to Dr. Richo, if any of these needs went unmet during childhood or adolescence, people may experience them as traumatic. This can alter a person's ability to form healthy relationships as adults. "These five As are a working definition of love. How do I know someone loves me? She pays attention rather than neglects me. She is able to show appropriate affection in accord to our ground rules of the relationship—this could be sexual or not. She values me just for who I am and accepts me as I am, rather than rejects certain parts of me. Finally, I still feel some wiggle room, that I'm able to make choices and honor my values, needs, and wishes that belong to me. I'm not giving up my independence. I'm folding it into an interdependence that allows me to still have autonomy while at the same time, carrying the commitment to our connection, which our relationship represents."[4]

In these scenarios, caregivers aren't the villains. They just didn't understand what their children needed, or if they did, for whatever reason, they couldn't meet it. "Some parents are better fits for some kids than they are for others," explained Jeff Ball, a psychologist.[5] "Well-meaning parents can be misattuned with their child, so that child will feel misunderstood and emotionally they feel like they've never gotten what they need, and that can create problems down the road. People tend to find similar relationships to their parental relationships, so they keep getting reinjured."[6]

To heal these wounds, you have to release the pain, and that can take many different forms, from breathwork to learning how to set boundaries that are right for you to forgiving yourself to doing inner-child work with a trained healer.

Traumatic Experiences Can Be Easy to Overlook

Whatever you experienced that was too much for your system to manage could have become a trauma. This makes for a very broad list. And while we have shied away from identifying specific traumas so far, we do want to mention a few common ones from childhood that the experts mentioned numerous times.

It's not that these events are worse than others. But some of the most common ones are what we can often push away. The acts and the trauma don't have to come from our parents either—they can happen at the hands of a loved one, a sibling, an authority figure, or a peer.

Let's take a closer look.

Sexual or Physical Abuse

Sexual or physical abuse is deeply traumatizing for most people who have lived through it—at any age. As a child, it's especially traumatic because it can take away any sense of self, and the child can feel so helpless over what's happening to them and what somebody is doing to them. It's the ultimate boundary violation and one of the hardest feelings to have.

Later in life, that feeling of helplessness remains under the surface, and it is so frightening that anytime you get close to it, it can feel like life and death—so many people will do almost anything to avoid experiencing that depth of pain again.

This can lead to many addictions, not just substance abuse or drugs, but to pornography or people—where someone else or something has to make you feel okay, because you don't know how to do it for yourself.

Neglect

Neglect has proven to be one of the biggest traumas, sometimes even more than physical abuse. Why do we put prisoners in isolation? Because it's damaging. Human beings are not meant to be left alone for long periods, especially little humans. We are social creatures. Kids need interaction from safe, loving, and caring adults, especially their parents and caregivers. When they're put in the basement, stuck in their room, and generally left alone, they're not being cared for—not physically, mentally, emotionally, or spiritually.

This has a huge impact on them. People who were raised in these environments often grow up with stories and beliefs like "nobody cares about me," or "I don't belong here," or "I don't matter at all," or "I'm not worthy of love," or "I'm not worthy of God/Divine's love." This last one doesn't have to be religious. It's the belief that no higher power would accept or love you, because if your parents can't love you, then how can spirit?

These devastating, heartbreaking beliefs can lead to low self-esteem and self-worth and unhealed wounds.

Abandonment

Many people who, between the ages of one and three, were left by their parents don't realize the trauma that they have endured. Even if they were left with a loving and caring grandparent, and even if they were reunited with their parents, it can still have an impact. Being torn away from a parent can affect your ability to trust others and to trust yourself. You may grow up feeling adrift in the world, where there's no place for you to be or call home.

This feeling can even come in infancy. Today we know more about how babies and little children sleep, their patterns, when to let them cry as a way to self-soothe, and how to sleep train. But back when many of us were being raised, that information wasn't as well known.

If you were constantly left to cry and nobody came for you, it could have felt like abandonment. We know that there are some "let the kid cry themselves to sleep" parenting styles. (You may even use that yourself.) There's controversy between both camps. There's no judgment here, and we're not wading into the "which is better" pool. All we can say is that some of the experts we spoke to believe that for some babies and little kids, letting them cry it out, whether during the day, at nap time, or at night, could have wounded them. A baby or little kid is not thinking rationally or logically—they can't do that developmentally. All they know is that something is off for them, and they feel terrified. They're using the only tool they have to get attention—crying—and it's not working.

And that can feel really frightening to a little person, and a sense of helplessness can ratchet up. Suddenly their systems are caught in a life-or-death struggle. And as we've said before, this can get hard-wired into our systems, showing up later through an inability to relax, where we feel that it's us against the world and there's no one we can rely on but ourselves.

Anger and Yelling in the Home

People lose their temper. Voices get raised. Fights between parents break out. What's the big deal? For some kids, it is a huge deal. Having one or two angry parents who yell a lot and who are irrationally angry often can have an incredible impact on a child's emotional stability and nervous system. Angry people have a way of saying hurtful, mean things, so it's easy for anger to escalate into belittlement or emotional abuse of their children.

These wounds run long and deep and can often get in the way of enjoying a healthy relationship with a romantic partner. Some people who come from such households may not be able to tolerate any raised voices. They may feel assaulted or threatened, triggering that fight, flight, or freeze response. And if one partner doesn't have the ability to sense when a disagreement, differing opinion, or conflict is nonthreatening, it can create problems in the relationship.

Gaslighting

As a child you may have said, "I feel scared," and instead of a parent validating that emotion, they might have said, "Oh, you're fine. There's nothing wrong." Or your caregiver may have insisted that you were making it up or were being too sensitive or dramatic. If you heard this a lot, it was a form of gaslighting, however unintentional. That's when someone makes us doubt our sanity and that what we see or feel isn't real.

When a parent tells a child that they cannot trust what their inner voice is telling them, they are telling them that they can't trust how they feel. When you start to question how you feel, you start to spin and judge yourself as wrong. Later in life this becomes a lived story. You tell yourself, "I'm too sensitive" or "I'm too dramatic."

When this happens, you can lose your connection to your intuition. You distrust yourself and stop believing in what you feel is right or wrong. You struggle to make decisions, set the right boundaries for yourself, and defend and protect yourself when it's called for.

This shows itself in relationships, especially difficult ones with a boss, a friend, or possibly your spouse or partner. You'll notice that something doesn't feel right, but then this little voice from childhood pops up, telling you, "You're wrong. You're making this up. Those red flags aren't real. You're being dramatic."

It becomes a vicious cycle where our adult lives become riddled with self-doubt, mistrust, and confusion. We can feel so "off" that we don't know who we are or what we believe, because in a very real sense, we don't.

Emotional Abuse

Were you ever made to feel worthless, no good, or rejected? Have you been teased, bullied, yelled at, or criticized repeatedly? If you are nodding along, then you were emotionally abused. Especially when our parents, loved ones, and people we trust put us down and make us feel worthless, it can be very traumatic.

For many kids, this trauma can destroy their sense of self and self-worth. They may think, *I'm not being good enough, strong enough, smart enough, thin enough, pretty or handsome enough, fast enough, or another (fill in the blank) enough.*

All trauma damages, yet emotional abuse is so deceptive. It burrows its way into our minds, poisoning us and how we see and feel about ourselves. It taints how we engage in relationships, the types of partners we feel we deserve, the kinds of jobs we accept, and the boundaries we place on how bosses, friends, co-workers, and other family members treat us.

❖

None of these traumas will go away without help. It takes time, commitment, patience, and a willingness to do the work to heal. There are so many resources, healing modalities, and therapies that can help you to close those wounds. By healing, these experiences don't magically disappear, but you can learn to put them in the past so that they no longer control your present or future.

Often buried within these traumas is so much intense pain that it can be difficult (sometimes even dangerous) to revisit and remember on your own. Please hear us when we say, you deserve and need a trusted guide and healer to help you on this journey. There is no shame in asking and seeking help.

The road to recovery is walked with many allies. You are not alone.

THE ROAD TO RECOVERY

Michael's doctor suspected that he may have had some hidden trauma that was getting in the way of his healing. With the encouragement of his wife and at his doctor's urging, Michael called and made an appointment with a psychotherapist his doctor recommended. Michael's expectations were pretty low—he didn't think there was anything in his past that needed addressing.

To his surprise, Michael liked the therapist and they didn't even talk about his past, not at first. They talked about how he managed stress and what felt stressful about his life, his worries, and his fears. These were topics he didn't think about too often, but voicing them out loud felt liberating.

Over time, his therapist recommended he try meditation, so he did, and Michael found he really liked that too (although at first, he could only meditate for a couple of minutes at a time). Over time, as he grew to trust his therapist more, he started talking more about his childhood.

Michael's parents had remained happily married, and they had never hit him, so Michael didn't think of his childhood as traumatic. However, he had lived in terror of his older brother, who would chase him with knives and baseball bats and beat him up after school before his parents got home from work.

When Michael tried to tell his parents, they would say, "Oh, that's boys being boys. Stop tattling on your brother, you're fine." When Michael tried to defend himself, they'd tell him to "be the bigger person," or "be the more mature one," or "don't let him bother you so much; that's how he is."

However, eventually his brother's torment got so bad, Michael's parents let Michael put a lock on his bedroom door. They told him to him to run upstairs quickly after school, lock himself in his room, and stay there until they get home. This made Michael uncomfortable, and it didn't always work because some days, his brother would get home before him and would be waiting in his bedroom for him. Because there was no safe space in his home for him, he became heavily involved in after-school sports and activities.

Michael had never learned how to relax, so overwork and chronic stress were the operating system that he carried into adulthood. His early experiences led him to shut off his emotions (they were too painful to confront at the time), and because his parents had told him this was no big deal in a form of gaslighting, he had believed them.

With his therapist's help and with a lot of patience and time, Michael slowly grieved for his younger self, for the boy who didn't get the protection he needed or deserved from his parents. He began to see how his boundaries were violated by his brother and that it was not okay how he had been treated.

As he gave his younger self a chance to speak and voiced what he had experienced to a safe and trusted ally, the underlying anger and impatience started to ebb. None of this happened instantly. It was a gradual journey to understand what had happened to him had been traumatic and to heal from that experience.

No one escapes childhood without some wounds. Left unhealed, we can carry them into adulthood, and they can get in the way of forming healthy connections to ourselves and loved ones. Michael reminded us how quickly we can bypass our childhood and early-adolescent experiences. It's easy to say, "leave the past in the past," but we never do until it's resolved and integrated. On your road to recovery, pausing to consider your history is worth it. It doesn't mean you have to force yourself to find a memory or seek to make your parents the villains of this story. Releasing trauma is about learning how to integrate and let go of painful experiences, whatever they were and whenever they occurred. Michael shows us that it's never too late to go back in time and heal the wounds of our past.

REFLECTIONS

Our childhoods are rife with potentially painful moments that need resolving. Take a few minutes and consider what memories immediately come to mind that may make you feel sad, angry, or anxious or that seem painful. There is no need to wade in too far here. You don't have to do anything with these memories now; your mission is to seek out where your blocks could be. You may want to make notes or keep a list of the painful memories that you may explore with a trusted ally later. Lastly, pay attention to any strong impression you had while you read this chapter and highlight any sections that you may want to revisit or to dig deeper for more information later.

SAGE WISDOM

"It's impossible to be born into this world and not have some kind of trauma that we have to heal and transcend."

—Marc David

CHAPTER 5

SOCIETAL TRAUMA

Nora's binge eating had returned. She had no idea why.

At 32, Nora had struggled with binge eating since college—it was nothing to finish a pint of ice cream and still want more. Raised by her grandmother, Nora's mother was an addict who was in and out of her daughter's life. Nora's grandmother was wonderful, but Nora was still battling with feelings of abandonment, betrayal, and unworthiness. Food had soothed her aching heart, and if she was honest, a little too much alcohol did too.

But in the last five years, Nora had worked very hard to heal her trauma and to overcome her dysregulated eating and drinking patterns. After trying a few therapists, she finally found a woman who had helped her to process the complicated emotions connected to her childhood. That's when Nora also adopted healthier lifestyle practices, including eating fresh foods, spending time in nature, journaling, taking up tai chi, and surrounding herself with quality people whom she trusted.

But then one day she slipped. It was at an airport on her way back from a trip to Cambodia, something she had planned for over a year. Her plane had been delayed, so she had gone to a bar, ordered two whiskeys, and then proceeded to buy cookies, chips, and candy bars from a vendor. She ate it all while at the gate.

She felt guilty and disgusted with herself, but she also told herself that it was just one slip. It had been a long eight days. She was exhausted, and she felt emotionally frayed.

But when Nora got home, the binge eating continued, along with more drinking and zoning out in front of the television when she got home from work. She found herself scrolling on her phone more too—it was the last thing she did before falling asleep and the first thing she did when she woke up.

Nora journaled regularly, and her entries were either filled with rage or depression. *The world is an ugly place*, she would write. *We're still committing terrible, atrocious acts against one another. What's the point of all of this? Will we ever learn?*

Nora knew her healthy lifestyle patterns were crumbling, and her behaviors and actions were unhealthy, but she didn't feel like her abandonment and betrayal issues with her mom had been triggered. She felt good in that part of her life, so she was confused.

Where were these intense emotions, the binge eating, and the self-destructive behaviors coming from, and more importantly, how could she stop them?

OUR TRIALS

There is an undercurrent of trauma pulsing through our society.

Most of us don't even recognize it because it's not a specific event that happens to us on an individual level. Instead it's *collective trauma*. Collective trauma is associated with a cataclysmic event that shatters the basic fabric of society, can generate horrific loss of life, and creates a crisis of meaning.[1]

We can point to the big events of the Holocaust, Vietnam War, 9/11, Hurricane Katrina, and scores of wars, genocide, and natural and manmade disasters. We'd expect anyone who has lived through any of these experiences to have some trauma that needs healing. But what's interesting is that you don't have to have a personal history with an event to be affected by it.

We are energetic beings, who are way more sensitive and connected to one another and this planet than we realize. The experts are finding that people can soak up trauma vicariously. You could have unhealed trauma that you absorb from visiting a place that you have seen, read about, or listened to on social media, the 24/7 news cycle, or the entertainment you consume. Trauma can get passed down through your parents, grandparents, and ancestors. You can even pick up trauma from the society and culture that you're born into, such as being a person of color in the United States or an immigrant.

Trauma coming from society is a sensitive topic.

We felt a little uneasy even writing this chapter and bringing up some of this trauma. But then we realized we cannot sugarcoat or ignore some of the darker parts of society and what it means to be a human being today. We have to keep having these conversations in order to get rid of stigmas and to heal. We are connected by our shared humanity, and a part of the experience of being human is to undergo trials and tribulations, to have painful experiences, and to learn how to heal our unresolved traumas.

Even amid universal experiences like a pandemic, no one will ever know exactly what your life has been like. But our hope is that you will see and feel the tapestry of human experiences as you walk through it, recognizing how collective moments and memories pass through time and impact so many people—possibly yourself—in ways that we have never imagined.

We know that talking about difficult and uncomfortable collective traumas can bring about a sense of despair. But we also know that when you allow healing into your life, you send ripples of love and connection into this world, affecting everyone who comes into your life in ways that you can't imagine.

Just as hurt people hurt people, healed people heal people.

As you journey through this chapter, be kind and compassionate to yourself if something pops up. You may be surprised at what you learn about yourself. And know that whatever discovery you make will become the first track you lay as you build a more loving, compassionate, healthier world—which is exactly what you, your children, grandchildren, and frankly, this entire world, need more than ever.

THE AWAKENINGS

Our Fear-Based Media and Entertainment Culture Can Traumatize

From social media to 24/7 news cycles to on-demand entertainment, we are constantly bombarded with information. Some of it is inspiring and hopeful, but a lot of it is trash and trouble.

As two guys immersed in media, we love the tools available to us. Social media, streaming devices, cell phones, tablets, computers, and television are incredible ways for us to connect with people. We get to share inspiring stories and wisdom from world-class leaders, and we get to fulfill our missions in life, which is to help more people heal. This is good stuff, and we're lucky to be alive at this moment in time.

But it would be foolish for us to ignore or downplay the dangers and harm these tools have wreaked on our society too.

Disturbing content disturbs the mind.

Our psyches and hearts are not built to withstand the nonstop onslaught of pictures and sounds of war, suffering, exploitation, and natural disasters. This content may overwhelm our capacity to cope, and sometimes we can experience it as traumatic.

This applies to television shows and movies. Have you noticed how, when you watch something scary, your heart pounds? That's your nervous system responding—as it should. Except that with the current media landscape, your nervous system is now being bombarded with external messages like "This world isn't safe. I'm not safe. Watch out. Hunker down. We've got to survive."

Sometimes what you see or hear is so overwhelming that it can shut you down. We're talking about becoming desensitized. Moderators on social media sites have reported psychological scars from the footage they witnessed.[2] It's so disturbing that some of the moderators have become numb to the graphic nature and feel "ground down" by it.[3]

And for all you parents out there, it's even more important for your kiddos. Little people are sponges. They're not just absorbing Mama and Papa's energy; they're taking in what you have on in the background. Kids are even more susceptible to this vicarious trauma from the media. They don't have the ability to separate what's happening in the world from what *could* happen to them. If you're someone who likes to have the news on in the background at night or in the morning, you may want to rethink what you expose the little ones to.

Violence and mayhem have become so prevalent that we have to become conscious consumers. Just like we are mindful about what we're eating and where our food comes from, we need to do the same with what we're watching and listening to.

The solution here isn't to go completely off the grid. We want you to be informed citizens, and you should know what's going on in the world and your community. While we cannot fully control our exposure or involvement with global trauma, to the extent we can, we should be mindful how much information we consume about it.

Consider what boundaries you can set to limit your intake of the trauma. There are so many ways to do this, and you're going to have to find the right balance between too much or too little. Maybe you only watch or read the news headlines for 20 minutes at lunch time. If you're someone who likes to start and end their day by scrolling through headlines, shift that. Start your morning with calm, centering practices that get you ready for the day and your energy pumping strong. End the day with a meditation, journaling, or something quiet and peaceful that signals to your body and mind that it's time to rest and unwind.

By having the news on constantly, it sends signals to your brain to always be in a state of high alert, threat, and anxiety. Shift to watching, listening, and reading material that inspires you and makes you feel good about yourself and life and hopeful about its possibilities. Consume more of the uplifting material that heals and teaches you, and you will be amazed at how it will shift your perspective on life, the world, and people.

You're Experiencing Intergenerational Trauma

Unhealed trauma can ripple through time, passed from one generation to the next.

This is the idea behind *intergenerational trauma*. What happens to one happens to others until someone decides to break the chain. For example, if your mother grew up with a cold, closed-off, and unaffectionate mother and it became an unhealed trauma for her, then she could have shown up for you as a cold, closed-off, unaffectionate mother.

In turn, that could have wounded you and left you with a "Little t" trauma that has impacted your life and how you relate to the world, yourself, and others.

How we engage with the world is all about intimacy. That may sound like a funny word to use, since we often associate that with our spouses or partners, but it's really about how we love, relate, and connect to people.

We first learn intimacy from our primary caregivers. Part of the reason so many people leave childhood with trauma is because the people raising and teaching us how to live and survive in this world are filled with so much unresolved pain that they can't teach us intimacy.

Stacie Aamon Yeldell, a board-certified music psychotherapist, shared a story about her relationship with her father that captures the essence of this idea. Stacie's father was an alcoholic, and she's done a lot of inner work to heal her wounds.

"Parents are only able to bring in what they've experienced themselves," said Stacie. "I had a conversation with my father, and he was saying, 'You know, I realize now how much my alcoholism affected my children, and I feel really guilty about that.' And I'm like, 'Well, look, I'm not going to absolve you of that, but I will say, if you're going to blame yourself, then you need to blame your mother, and your mother's mother. You're going to have to bring everybody into the room, because you only acted based on what your experience of loving intimacy and parenting was based upon, and that was how your mother showed up for you."[4]

The only way the chain of intergenerational pain breaks is if someone consciously chooses to change the cycle. Sometimes that happens when a parent decides to raise their child the opposite way from how they were raised. For example, if a man grew up with a very strict and rigid dad, then he may consciously decide to be the opposite with his own children.

Choosing to engage differently with the world and our children is only part of the equation. If there are still wounds unhealed from how you were raised, they will need healing. The good news is that we're living during a time where talking about our traumas and healing from them is more accepted than ever.

More people are consciously choosing to go inward, to get to know themselves and peer into the dark corners to say, "Hey, I want to heal from my traumas. I am willing to go on this journey and to do the work so I don't have to live in this pain anymore or pass it along to my children or grandchildren."

By going to therapy and doing that inner work on ourselves, we can begin unpacking the cycles of trauma and breaking them so that we don't carry these patterns forward with future generations.

We are blessed with so many different healing modalities and therapies. From working with a therapist to an energy healer to a shaman in South America to a massage or body work specialist, we have choices like never before. And it's never been easier to try a therapy, see if it works, and then move on, or to explore one form for a few months and then move on to something else when it's time to expand and evolve.

What it takes is a willingness and desire to heal—which we know you already have.

Historical Trauma May Haunt You

When we think of trauma, we think of a very specific event or experience that happened *directly* to us. However, there's another form of trauma that doesn't get as much airtime but can have just as big an impact on how we move through the world, and it's called *historical trauma*. This is "the complex and collective trauma experience that happens to a group of people who share an identity, affiliation or circumstance that happens over time and across generations."[5]

The term came from Dr. Maria Yellow Horse Brave Heart, whose interest in the subject came from her research and work with the Lakota tribe and her own experiences being Native. "I had a sense of carrying grief that was larger than myself and my own community," said Brave Heart. "I made a conscious connection that American Indians are survivors and that we share some things in common with Jewish Holocaust communities."[6]

Brave Heart described the trauma as the result of centuries of abuses, including the separation of families and forced assimilation of Native children into boarding schools.[7] In her research, she found that people can experience guilt, depression, PTSD symptoms, physical symptoms, psychic numbing, anger, suicidal ideation, and a fixation to the trauma.[8]

Today historical trauma is applied to many indigenous and minority groups who have suffered and shared a history of oppression, victimization, or massive group trauma exposure.[9] Some examples include racism and slavery, forced migration such as people fleeing from war-torn countries, colonization of indigenous people, descendants of Holocaust survivors, and survivors of genocide.

And before we go further, let's pause and recognize that historical trauma is a *heavy subject.*

These are often dark acts that we as a society don't want to talk about, and often survivors don't either. But the experiences continue to haunt generations in very real emotional, spiritual, psychological, and physical ways. Part of healing is acknowledging the pain and validating what we feel because of these experiences.

These experiences are not often left in the past, and they reverberate into the present. If we look closely at the United States, we can see this playing out with race issues. Look at the historical and collective trauma that Black people and people of color experience with police shootings and brutality and economic and housing opportunities. Look at the experiences of Native peoples and the extreme rates of poverty, depression, violence, and suicide that are being experienced on reservations today. Look at immigrants from all over the world who were forced to flee because of political or social instability and unrest, who face discrimination and uncertainty. Look at the experiences of women who continue to fight for equal pay, rights, and opportunities in the workforce as men—and society at large.

Gwen Dittmar, M.S., a life coach and healer, stated, "I work with female executives, and they'll tell me they know deep down the company shouldn't do that marketing plan, but they don't have the data to back it up. They don't bring it up in a meeting because they're afraid they'll be told they're crazy or something's wrong with them or they're being difficult. This dates back to a collective trauma where women were told 'they're crazy,' or 'hysterical,' or 'overly emotional' or 'sensitive.'[10]

"Look at ancient times, and women were the ones who were intuitive and connected to source. They felt into everything and knew what was aligned and not. Somewhere, whether you want to say it was the patriarchy or the agricultural or industrial revolutions, but somewhere women's intuition was viewed as crazy. This is a trauma I see in a lot of women."[11]

Look at the experiences of Middle Easterners and people of the Islamic faith. After 9/11, many of them faced racism and hate just because they may have shared an ethnicity or religion with the terrorists. People have been villainized and discriminated against for nothing.

When we really stop to look at our society, it's heartbreaking. There are instances of historical trauma everywhere, and these moments can leave scars. They leave traces on our souls in ways that we don't understand, and they can be so subtle that we don't even realize they exist.

Healing from these wounds can take time. It's not always easy to uncover them, but with some patience and the right healers and therapists, you can begin to work through your beliefs and wounds connected to the past.

There are healers and therapists who specialize in historical trauma, so if discussing it just now felt like you were finally seen for the first time or you felt a little shiver, then this might be worth investigating. If you've struggled to identify *where* your trauma comes from, but you know deep in your soul that something is off, this might be it.

Anything goes, and everything is worth investigating if it can help restore your center and return you to a state of balance and harmony.

Suicide Affects More People than We Realize

Suicide is the quiet epidemic that our society avoids discussing even more than trauma in general.

According to the World Health Organization, one person dies by suicide every 40 seconds.[12] In young people ages 15–19, it is the second leading cause of death.[13] In the United States, one person dies by suicide every 11 minutes.[14] And these numbers don't take into consideration the millions of people who seriously think about taking their lives, make a plan, and attempt it.

It's heartbreaking to live through an experience where a parent, spouse, significant other, sibling, child, close friend, co-worker, or boss dies by suicide.

The loss of a loved one to suicide is traumatic, and it's often made worse by cultural and societal taboos and stigmas. Just talking about death is hard in many cultures, especially in the West. But then you add in certain cultural and religious beliefs that suicide is a sin, and it makes it harder to address this issue in a meaningful and healing way.

As a society, we dislike talking about many of the underlying issues that can lead to someone dying by suicide. In the United States, some have a belief that most people who die by suicide have mental health issues, but that's not always the case. According to the CDC, 54 percent of people who died by suicide *did not* have an underlying mental health issue.[15]

We are living in a time when many people feel left out by society. There can be issues and unhealed trauma around poverty, race, ethnicity, marginalization. We also know that people who have endured more adverse childhood experiences and are veterans are at a higher risk for suicide.

When we asked the experts what was going on, the same answer appeared: pain. More precisely, the fact that we don't know how to experience it.

"We aren't taught that pain is actually okay, and a healthy, normal, and natural part of being alive," explained Dr. Sam Rader, a psychologist. "We're shown that the second you start to feel a headache, you should pop an aspirin, and we're told that life is about being happy—just be happy, always.[16]

"We're not taught the beauty and power and the sacredness and the natural illness of wrestling with pain, emotional and physical. So when we feel pain that is so great, we think it's wrong to feel that, and we don't know how to make use of it. If we go into the heart of pain, there's usually quite a jewel there that can help us blossom into more of who we really are, but instead we try to resist the pain or get rid of it."[17]

When we don't experience pain after an event, it creates trauma. And when the trauma goes on for so long, and it's so deep, and more traumas pile up, it can feel like too large of a burden to bear.

Rader's talking about what happens after a trauma, but there are layers of trauma that get added directly and vicariously. "There is a lot of turmoil going on throughout the world that people are watching or listening to," explained Dr. Mark L. Gordon.[18] "It can take longer for us to feel the effects of world or national stress, but you add that to our emotional stress, mental stress, taking certain drugs, medication, drinking alcohol, not eating correctly, not getting enough physical activity, and it generates stress, and all these inflammatory chemicals are unleashed. Inflammation disrupts the functioning of the brain. Depending upon how susceptible you are, it can generate things like mood change, personality change, depression, and suicide ideation.

"It comes to a point where someone can't intellectually or logically analyze what's going on and know that this moment is passing. They're so overwhelmed with the information that is so negative or so challenging that they end up taking their own life."

We can't talk about suicide without talking about what's happening to teens today either. Suicides in the United States among teens is on the rise.[19] It is the second leading cause of death for young people between the ages of 15 and 24, and this is true for all races and ethnicities.[20] Between 2007 and 2017, the rate of suicides increased by a staggering 56 percent.[21]

Researchers and the experts we spoke to say there is still so much to learn and understand about what's happening to our youth. But we don't think it's a coincidence that during that 10-year period, our lives moved online in ways we've never experienced. This was the dawn of social media, of everyone carrying cell phones, of being "on" 24/7. Look at cyber bullying and the very real toll that is taking on our youth—and, let's be real, on everyone.

The internet and social media have afforded us incredible ways to connect with each other—but it's also driven us apart. People can be nasty to each other. They can make incredibly harmful and hurtful comments—some of which are extremely threatening. The more visible you are online, the more you become a target for this abuse, especially if you're a woman.

There are ugly truths about our society, and the wounds people collect can add up to the point where it's just too much.

Suicide is a very complex topic. No one can make sense of painful, unhealed trauma—or even the societal ones hitting us daily—alone. There is a time and place to be fiercely independent and self-reliant. Dealing with pain and trauma—and suicide—is not it.

You need guides and healers who can help you break down these personal and societal traumas into small enough pieces that you can digest and absorb.

If you are experiencing any ideas of suicide, please seek help. If it's an emergency, you can call a suicide hotline and speak with a trained professional. You can reach out to your therapist, doctor, or another trained professional who can help you work through your emotions and whatever traumas may be coming up.

Also, as we've mentioned earlier, science and modern medicine are finding connections between TBIs and brain inflammation, and symptoms of PTSD, suicide ideation, mood disorders, anxiety, and depression. So, if you're experiencing suicide ideation, it might be worth looking into whether you're experiencing a TBI or hormonal or chemical imbalances.

And if you've experienced the loss of someone you love from suicide, please seek help too. That's a very real, painful experience, and there are specialists in the healing world who can help you work through that pain.

There are ways through these traumatic mazes, and so many people are waiting and wanting to help you. Wherever you are right now, please keep going. The world needs you.

THE ROAD TO RECOVERY

After about a month, Nora knew she needed to see her therapist more consistently instead of the sporadic appointments that she had been having. It took a few visits, but Nora eventually connected the dots, and they led her to her trip to Cambodia.

Nora visited the Killing Fields, where millions of people died and families were torn apart because of genocide under the Khmer Rouge regime. Nora had been wholly unprepared for the distinct energy of death and suffering. As she walked slowly across the land, she felt something, but she didn't have words to describe or understand what it was.

For the rest of her trip, her thoughts drifted to the memorials, and she was preoccupied by thoughts of how unfair the world is and how terrible people are.

Then when she was in the airport, the television above her showed a news story on Syria, where the reporter was talking to refugees and asking them to share their experiences.

As Nora recounted her experience in Cambodia with her therapist, Nora's voice became angry and her movements animated until she eventually deflated. Visiting the Killing Fields in Cambodia had deeply affected her, and she hadn't processed it or made sense of it. Then when she saw the news, it was too much negativity. The binge eating and drinking were reactions to the intense emotions that she had vicariously experienced on her vacation.

Nora's therapist explained how difficult it can be to watch or be present for an experience while staying removed from it. Before Nora's next appointment, her therapist suggested that she track how much time she spent watching or reading the news, using social media, and consuming violent, disturbing, or upsetting content on a movie or television show. In one week, Nora averaged about 4–5 hours a day—which surprised her too.

She never noticed how negative and violent, and, frankly, disturbing her viewing habits were (Nora's certainly not alone there).

As an experiment, Nora's therapist told her to cut her viewing time at least in half and that she should bookend her days reading something uplifting, meditating, or doing something that was peaceful and relaxing to her nervous system. Nora agreed, and after one week she said she already felt lighter and less sad and angry.

Nora stuck with this practice and with the help of her therapist decided to focus on how she could bring more of her values of fairness and justice into the world. Every day she set an intention to show acts of kindness like holding the door open for someone, looking people in their eyes and offering a genuine smile, or speaking up for a co-worker at the office.

Everywhere she went, she would look for these opportunities to sync her actions with the world she wanted to live in. That was very empowering for Nora, and it inspired her to also look for ways she could volunteer in her community. She felt passionate about social justice issues, so she looked for nonprofits and organizations that needed extra help—this helped to shift her worldview from a negative, dark place to one that was positive and focused on making a difference for the better.

Finally, Nora realized that she's very sensitive to the world and people around her. She needed more outlets to help her process her experiences in life and to keep building her resiliency. She decided to try joining a group art therapy program that met once a week on Wednesday nights. She *loved* it. It was the perfect mix of creative expression and a chance to connect with people in a community and healing situation.

Today, Nora realizes that healing trauma is not a quick fix; it's something that she's committed to for the rest of her life.

Trauma can surprise us. We think we've released it only to experience it reawakening, possibly triggered by a current event. What inspired us about Nora's story was how in tune she was with her body and its habits. She knew she had slipped into some unhealthy behaviors, even if she didn't know why, so she sought help. By working with trusted allies, Nora discovered that it wasn't just one traumatic event, it was the combination of visiting the Killing Fields mixed with consuming too much negative content that had started the spiral. Her road to recovery became a combination of remedies.

You may not know where your trauma is coming from, and that's okay. The key is to first recognize that something is off in your life, then to begin taking actions toward releasing the pain. These don't have to be giant leaps forward either. Right now, you can take a quick content inventory in what you're consuming and commit to cutting it in half, or at least by 25 percent. Or maybe you pause and reflect on whether intergenerational or historical trauma could have a hook in you, and from there you look for a trauma-informed therapist who may have experience working with patients on these subjects (you can always ask them point-blank if they have).

There are so many paths to releasing trauma, but you can't let go of something you aren't aware of. So be mindful of how you're living. Pay attention if something feels off in your life or if you have habits that you'd like to change. By noticing this, you open the door to your healing.

REFLECTIONS

It's easy for us to disregard what's happening globally and its effects on us. But those are real. Take a couple of minutes and consider whether you have been affected by a societal trauma. Listen to how your body reacted as you read through this chapter. Did you feel a pit in your stomach? Did you get shivers or goose bumps? Did your hands start sweating? Did you have a strong emotional reaction like tears that formed, or did you feel angry? These may be signs that societal trauma has hooked into you. Write down any reactions so that when it is time to dive into remedies and treatments, you will know what you're releasing.

SAGE WISDOM

"If we can't talk about problems, we can't see them, and if we can't see them, we can't solve them."

—Laura Kalmes

CHAPTER 6

SPIRITUAL TRAUMA

Sarah knew she needed help.

Until she was 21 years old, Sarah had been opposed to drinking and partying. Growing up in a strict Catholic home, her parents instilled in her strong beliefs around sinning and amoral behaviors. Her mother especially didn't want Sarah having a "child out of wedlock" or drinking, which she thought could lead to "promiscuity."

Legally, Sarah could drink now, and her friends convinced her to one night. It felt like a revelation. *Oh, wow, this is what I've been missing*, she thought.

Sarah had always felt anxious and nervous, especially around other people. She was quiet and shy. But alcohol calmed her. It took away her painful insecurities. It made it easier to go out and meet people, let loose, and relax even when she was alone. When she drank, she got more attention from the guys too. Suddenly, Sarah was having one-night stands and casually dating.

Alcohol also fueled her creativity. As an artist and writer, she felt like she was settling into the "artist lifestyle" and becoming a new person. During the day, she worked as a secretary in a dentist's office; at night, Sarah the artist came alive, drinking, partying, having sex, and creating.

One night, she was out late drinking with a friend. When she got to her door, she couldn't get her key into the lock. That's when two men surprised her from behind, beat her up, and stole her purse. Eventually, she picked herself up, walked into the apartment, got into the shower, and went to bed. The only person she told was her roommate.

Flashbacks to this robbery started almost immediately. Sarah felt panic and fear course through her body every time she stepped outside. To blunt the intensity of emotions and memories, Sarah turned to alcohol, drinking to numb and forget. But this time it made her feel worse. She stopped showing up to work. She struggled to get out of bed.

She knew she was spiraling down, but she didn't know how to pull herself up. One night, Sarah's roommate walked into her room and told her gently, "I think you need help, not just for the assault, but it seems like there's something deeper on going."

Something about the way her roommate spoke to her, mixed with her trauma, broke through for her. Sarah agreed that she needed help in order to find what was buried under the alcohol.

OUR TRIALS

In times of crisis, what do many of us do? We pray for help, guidance, and easing of our pain and suffering. We turn to God in whatever form feels true to us—Allah, the Divine, the Universe, All-That-Is, the Goddess, Shiva, Krishna, the Great Spirit—to heal.

We pray to heal, but what happens when our trauma comes from our religious and spiritual life?

Similar to societal trauma, a lot of people don't realize how deeply their religious and spiritual communities have affected them. Like all traumas, this one covers a lot of ground. It includes sexual, physical, emotional abuse from religious and spiritual leaders, such as that from the priest and clerical sex abuse scandals. It can come from feeling abandoned and rejected by our faith communities when we do something "wrong" or sinful in their eyes, including getting divorced, being in a same-sex relationship, or losing a loved one to suicide.

Then there's the secondary spiritual trauma we can experience after a "Big T" or "Little t" event. By its nature, trauma leaves us feeling disconnected from ourselves and from the Divine. So, not only do we have to heal the initial trauma, we have to heal our connection to spirit too.

When we really start examining spiritual trauma, we realize it's a giant knot of conflicting and complicated emotions and layered experiences. On top of that, so many of us lack the language to even understand or describe what we're feeling or thinking.

To untangle this massive trauma knot, we have to take it one thread at a time.

So, on this leg of our journey, we're going to give you the insights and words to better understand what could be going on inside you. We'll explore how spiritual trauma might show itself in your life, from issues with trust and faith, to false beliefs about yourself and the world, to living without a purpose or meaning.

Just as spiritual trauma might be the source of your wounds, religious and spiritual communities can also be your path to healing and recovery. No, your spiritual practice probably won't look the same as before. You may never return to the same faith. You might find a different one with a new community. Maybe you connect to the Divine in all life, experiencing the beauty in this world without ever stepping into a place of worship. And if you need to cool it for a time with religion, spirituality, and faith, that works too.

It's cliché, we know, but there are so many paths up this mountain. We only sincerely hope that you take the journey to rediscovering your connection to spirit. We'd go so far as to say that we all need some connection to something bigger than ourselves. It's a primary source of resilience.

In Viktor Frankl's book *Man's Search for Meaning*, he writes about what it was like for him living and surviving in a concentration camp during the Holocaust. He explained how his spiritual connection and faith were sources of comfort, and that those who survived the atrocities were the ones who held on to their beliefs too. Despite the horrors he and others endured, kindness, compassionate, generous people still existed. He could see the best of humanity and our religious and spiritual teachings through the cruelty.

Love for one another lies at the core of most organized religions. It's just that humankind has co-opted, misinterpreted, and used these teachings for power and greed, and that's created a lot of harm.

No matter what spiritual trauma you've endured, there is still so much love and compassion and such grace and beauty in this world—even if it's a little hard to access right now. If you can put aside the "man-made" rules and religious interpretations, then you're likely to find awe, connection, faith, and love in a spiritual practice.

Whenever you're ready to go on this particular quest, remember that how you return to your connection with the Divine and what it looks like don't matter. There is no right religion—there never has been—and there is no right way to find your way to the Divine, God, the Universe, or whatever or whomever you want to call it.

You get to choose your path.

Over time, it's likely to change and evolve, just as you do. So whatever road you decide to walk on, that's the right one. Trust it.

And when it comes to healing spiritual trauma, give yourself time. Explore at your own pace, and be forgiving of yourself. Finding harmony between divinity and humanity is tough stuff. There are no easy answers, and there will be many dark nights of the soul. But we have faith in you. At our core, we're all pilgrims and seekers on this journey together. Just be willing to ask the questions, face the truth of your experiences, and keep searching for answers.

Embrace curiosity as you go on this journey, and be willing to let *faith find you.* Let your heart lead the way, especially for this particular path.

THE AWAKENINGS

Your Trust and Faith Have Been Shattered

Spiritual trauma can shatter our worldview, causing us to lose trust and faith in everything and everyone, including ourselves. This has to do with the role that our religion and faith often play in our lives. Let's take a quick look at what our spiritual communities have offered us.

Sanctuary. Our spiritual traditions and religions are supposed to be physical places we go to feel connected and safe. Throughout history, churches and places of worship were supposed to be safe havens for people to rest, heal, and live without fear for their safety or lives.

Knowledge. Teachings and knowledge passed to us from sacred books explore morals and values, what's right versus wrong, how to see ourselves and others, and how to live our lives.

Role models and leaders. Religious leaders and people who hold positions of power and authority interpret these sacred texts, deliver sermons, and pass on to us the lessons of how to live in accordance with our religious and spiritual laws. They are role models, and we look to them to shepherd us through this physical world.

Connection to a higher power. At the core of religion rests a belief in divinity, a supreme being that sits at the center of our beliefs. We pray to this entity, seeking guidance and safety and care from them. We turn to our religion and spirituality to feel connected to something bigger than ourselves, find a sense of belonging and acceptance, and know that there is more to life than what we may see.

Belonging and support. For many people, their church, synagogue, or mosque is their family. It's their community and place where they're supported during times of need and struggle. For a lot of people, their religious and spiritual lives began as children in the places their parents worshipped. In some households, there's no separation between their immediate family and their religious or spiritual community.

"What can come out of trauma is a sense of 'I must not be okay because God let this happen to me' or 'God made this happen to me' or 'God is not okay because this happened to me' or 'the universe isn't okay because this isn't what was supposed to happen' or 'I just don't know who's wrong, me or God or the universe?'" explained Rabbi Arielle Hanien.[1] "It can be really hard to orient, particularly when what gave us a sense of the universe or a place in it or whom we could trust, human or not, is the same thing that caused the pain."[2]

When it comes to restoring trust and faith, it can take a long time, and it's very much an inward, reflective journey. It requires establishing new worldviews and stories, finding and setting boundaries that are right for us, discerning and allowing the right people—those who are safe and trustworthy—into our lives, coming to terms with what this world is and isn't, and dealing with feeling betrayed and grieving.

You may not return to your original religion. Perhaps your road to recovery comes from learning about others or finding a community that feels more authentic to you. Sometimes the journey is about exploring spirituality in your own way through nature, New Age practices, or ancient indigenous ones. Sometimes it's working through your complicated emotions with a therapist and healer (the go-to for healing trauma). Often, it's a combination of all of the above.

While ultimately you have to find the path that suits you best, we can tell you that most of the experts we spoke to said having a spiritual practice creates a strong foundation for recovery and resiliency. While we'd never say, "You must have one," we strongly advise you to undertake the journey. If you can find peace in your beliefs and a connection to a higher power, it can help you overcome so much in your life—especially in making peace with yourself, your life, and your trauma.

You May Be Living with False Beliefs

Religious narratives are ancient. They're older than anyone living can remember. That means they're open for interpretation, though it's not often presented that way to us. They're delivered as truth, fact, and being objective.

But the real truth is these meanings and conclusions come from our religious and spiritual leaders who are human beings. They're flawed, imperfect, and they make mistakes. Religion and spiritual teachings aren't usually the problem. It's the people running the show, telling the stories, and crafting the meaning that are. And they may be confused, embittered, judgmental, or filled with righteousness to the point of harm.

The form this trauma takes is in the false beliefs we form about ourselves, other people, the world, and the Divine. Beliefs are thorny. They're formed at an unconscious level, and we act them out without realizing what we're doing since we don't even know they exist.

There are a multitude of damaging messages and false beliefs that get funneled to us. We'll be highlighting some of the most common and traumatic ones that can leave us feeling riddled with shame, guilt, self-loathing, anger, rage, and self-doubt. We're hauling these stories out from the darkness, so you can see them clearly. Learn to recognize them so you can start to rewrite your story.

Your natural instincts are wrong

Some teachings judge our natural wants and desires for pleasure— be it sex, food, money—as bad and wrong. In many religions, it's not about finding balance; it's about shutting off and controlling the impulse. Too much of anything is indeed harmful, but balance and moderation are the keys to creating a healthy relationship with anything in life.

If you suppress your emotions, sexuality, or desires, you may become controlling, filled with fear, or shut off entirely from your emotions and desires. We're talking no sense of pleasure or pain, no tears, nothing.

Your behaviors may even lean in the other direction. You may use drugs, alcohol, or sex as coping mechanisms or outlets for expressing yourself. This can lead to addictions, where nothing you do really changes you. It just causes more trauma as you get further from yourself.

Do you know what else is instinctive? Your intuition. When you're taught to control your instincts, then you learn to mistrust your inner voice. Silencing or ignoring your inner voice is traumatic, and it can remove one of the most important censors you have helping you to navigate the world.

You should feel good about feeling bad

Martyrdom litters many Christian traditions. Think Christ sacrificing himself on the cross for humankind. These stories can teach you that sacrificing yourself and giving up your needs and wants for someone else are what make you a "good person." And you may feel that if you dare to ask for something, then you're a "bad person."

This creates a distorted view for yourself because you learn to associate what feels good with being bad, and what feels bad with being good. Living with this belief system can create a lot of pain in your relationships. You may get involved with someone who never considers your needs or wants. Or you may put up with a job or career that's unsatisfying, but you figure, "that's my lot in life," so you stick with it.

You may also experience the reverse too. You may become so filled with anger, bitterness, and resentment about a world that exploits you and doesn't seem to care about you. Sometimes that anger can turn into rage that you put into the world.

That's confusing, right? It's mind-boggling and harmful. As an adult, you have to retrain and relearn that what feels good is good, and that what feels bad is bad.

You should never acknowledge some topics and "sins"

Religions and spiritual communities can ignore the complexities of life. Being a human is messy, unpredictable, and uncertain. We need support through these times and compassion for when we make mistakes or something doesn't turn out the way we had expected. We need to know that everything is still okay, that we're okay.

Some spiritual practices don't offer this, making us feel abandoned, unsupported, and ashamed. Take suicide for example. Many people feel they can't talk about suicide because of their religion's belief that it is a sin and unacceptable. This was Dr. Ruchira Densert's story. Dr. Densert's ex-husband died by suicide three days before their son turned 12 (their daughter was 10 at the time). "I was a psychiatrist. It was my job to help people, to keep them from getting to that point, and the sense of guilt and shame that came from that . . . it's been difficult to talk about."[3]

Some of that difficulty comes from her religious upbringing and the beliefs her mother still has. Dr. Densert was born in India, and the region her mother is from believes that if someone dies by suicide, then for their next seven lifetimes, they will be reincarnated as a bird. Suicide is unacceptable, so Dr. Densert hasn't been able to turn to her mother for support. They haven't spoken about her ex-husband's death at all. This has made the trauma all the more painful because it has created isolation.

It's a similar story around divorce. Dr. Debi Silber, a transformational psychologist, said that many of her clients have stayed in marriages after being betrayed because of religious teachings. "According to their religion, they are not supposed to divorce," said Dr. Silber. "They were grappling with understanding, 'How could my religion want me to stay in something that is so bad, so wrong, and that has me feeling horrible about myself, and that has shattered any sense of worthiness?' They [her clients] just couldn't make sense of their religion."[4]

Both examples highlight the complexity of spiritual trauma. Instead of our religious and spiritual beliefs supporting and strengthening our resolve during times of strife and heartache, they can make the pain—and trauma—worse.

God's love is conditional

Many of our religions teach us that our higher power is harsh and judgmental. You better be "good" if you want to be loved and allowed into heaven.

You want to talk about traumatizing a kid, here it is. From day one, we're told, "You better shape up and get in line, because if you don't, here's your one-way ticket to fire and brimstone, and eternal damnation." Instead of creating and nurturing our relationship with the divine as a source of love and compassion and support, the divine becomes threatening. We're only safe with our higher power some of the time, and our needs become conditional. We have to be "good," otherwise, no love for us.

In these teachings, we also learn that the higher power only works for some people. Being gay can sometimes be a double whammy of trauma. Many people face being rejected and hurt by their families, who can't or won't accept their sexuality for their own personal reasons. Then you layer on rejection from their church and God, and now we're talking abandonment and the magnification of trauma by your support systems and the places and people who were supposed to love and support you unconditionally.

❖

The good news is that it's never too late to rewrite your spiritual story or to form a healthier connection to the Divine that's based on love, compassion, forgiveness, and safety, and all that is right in this world.

It might be that you have to relearn how to connect to spirit, to see the Divinity as merciful, benevolent, filled with grace, and love. Even if you don't have a connection, you can learn it. Anybody at any time in their lives can learn how to connect to spirit in a way that feels right to them.

"When I work with people who have had spiritual abuse, they don't have to be open to whatever concept of God they were taught," shared psychologist Margaret Paul, Ph.D. "They can open to any concept, being, angel, higher self—anything that they can visualize as kind, caring, wise, powerful, and compassionate."[5]

As Dr. Paul shared, she helps people move beyond their old beliefs and concepts of God until they get to a point where they really believe and feel that the universe is love, that spirit is love, that God is love.

Healing these false beliefs can happen. It takes time, patience, consistency, and working with someone you trust and who will hear and see you as the amazing person and being that you are and always have been.

There's Little to No Connection to Your Purpose

Do you know your purpose? Do you feel connected to it? Are you living it?

Having nothing to live for and no purpose for being can be traumatic. We need a purpose that gives us meaning and fulfilment—a mission that's our true soul food. Without it, we feel adrift and disconnected from the world, our loved ones, and ourselves.

And what about your community—your friends, family, and support network? Do you have people in your life who support, love, respect, and care for you? The trauma of being alone and feeling lonely doesn't get enough airtime, but a number of the experts we spoke to mentioned it. Feeling lonely is one of the most significant risk factors for dying young and for getting sick.[6]

We need human connections, a place to belong, and meaning and purpose for our lives and time on earth. When we're missing any of these pieces, we are wounded. Left unattended, this pain will show up in our bodies. "The number one indicator of whether somebody is going to have low back pain is whether they are satisfied with the work they're doing every day," said Dr. Patrick Gentempo, DC.[7] "In essence, are you satisfied with your purpose in life? Do you feel like you're getting up every day and you have purpose, or are you going to a job that you don't find any purpose in? Low back pain is more of a psycho-emotional issue than it is a physical or mechanical."[8]

So, let's reflect on how you're living. Are you happy? Are you engaged? If money was no object, what would you do with your time and energy? What are your strengths? What skills do you have that come naturally and easily and that you like using? Or imagine yourself on your death bed where the Divine will grant you one last wish. What would it be?

This isn't necessarily about what you feel passionate about. Passions flare and fade. This is about connecting to your spirit and knowing *this* is what you were put on earth to do and who you were born to be.

We don't have the answers for you, and no expert can tell you how to live your purpose and find meaning. That's for you to find, but please know that you can do it. The answers are out there. Go on that quest and stick with it until you find what you're looking for.

For both of us, we know our mission is to help people heal. Every day, we work hard to help people cut through all the noise, reconnect to their internal compass, and get their systems aligned.

When you *know* it's right, everything aligns and you feel it in your gut. When you have unresolved trauma, this can be hard to recognize. Trauma causes our internal compasses to spin wildly, so we can't tell true north from due south. But as you heal, your instinct and connection to yourself will return. It may take a lot of practice and time to learn how to trust yourself, but stick with it.

It will come back.

THE ROAD TO RECOVERY

Sarah's road to recovery has been a long and winding one. It started with a couple of years of therapy to deal with the assault and her PTSD reactions. During this time, Sarah had a string of failed relationships, was fired from her job, and struggled to make money with her art. She also continued to drink, and it was her therapist who helped her realize that getting sober might be the best solution.

So Sarah began her sobriety journey. She joined a 12-step program and found a supportive and encouraging community of people who understood her, and they changed the course of her life. Once sober, she felt strong enough to unravel and unwind the origins of her anxiety and what had driven her to drink in the first place.

Sarah grew up with a very strict, Catholic upbringing. She was taught to fear sex and anything remotely sensual and that she would go to hell if she sinned. She didn't want to disappoint her parents, the church, or God, so she didn't drink, party, or "let loose" at all.

Sarah was highly sensitive too. She seemed to feel more than most people, but she was taught not to show her emotions and to keep them inside and "suffer in silence." She never learned how to process or deal with her emotions, or even what were healthy outlets for them. She also had a hard time connecting with people. Her parents moved their family a lot, so making friends was hard. To deal with life, Sarah would escape into her mind.

By the time she hit her adult years, she was ready to break free and rebel from the controlled upbringing that she was raised in. Drinking and sex were her outlets to feel alive and find her place in the world. She had created her own identity as a suffering artist, and she had enjoyed keeping her life a secret from her parents—they never knew the extent of her drinking or partying (they don't to this day).

Sarah had to find a way to authentically connect to herself, and in many ways, find herself for the first time. It has taken time, but it's been a journey she's committed to with her heart and soul. She spent a few years as an atheist, went to Baptist, Methodist, and Episcopalian churches, and she explored Judaism, Buddhism, and Shamanic healing, which helped her learn how to feel more grounded in life. Right now, she does not identify with the Catholic Church or any organized religion.

One of the most important practices and healing modalities on her journey has been her art. Sarah went back to school for training in expressive arts therapy, which included a dance component that has given her a new level of understanding in her body. Through art, she's found a means of expression for her emotions and identity and a way to connect to spirit in a healthy way.

The religions that we're exposed to and brought up in influence us in ways that we may not realize. Even if we've "left the church," its teachings may have stayed with us. Until we do the work to unwind any false beliefs that got programmed, we may never be free. What strikes us as extraordinary, though, is how many people we spoke to who were like Sarah. They have struggled mightily to reconcile religion with their connection to God, spirit, and themselves, but it has been a journey worth taking. By understanding their relationship with their religious upbringing, it's given them the opportunity to find their own path to God and a deeper connection to spirit and to who they are.

That's the heart of Sarah's story. Through her traumas, she's discovered herself and found a deeper connection to spirit. She's found her way, one step at a time, and that's the lesson we can all take. That as we journey toward our traumas and find ways to release them and integrate them into our being, we discover ourselves and create a relationship with spirit that is right for us.

REFLECTIONS

Could your trauma be connected to religion? Could an early teaching or specific upbringing have left an imprint on you? Did you lose faith in a higher power along the way? Do you feel connected to the Divine, God, or a higher power? Do you have a sense of purpose in the world? These are questions to sit in quiet contemplation with, acknowledging any links to a traumatic experience. Think about what your early life was like and whether you grew up in a religious household. If you did, think about what, if any, messages or lessons you picked up from it and whether it may be getting in the way of your life now. If you had a strong emotional reaction to anything in this chapter, then note that too. Religious trauma can be obvious (clergy abuse) or subtle (religious teachings that you were raised with).

SAGE WISDOM

"I had the good fortune to be born in a war. Why good fortune? I don't wish it on anybody, but I saw what happens when people don't cultivate life and awareness and peace, and that can cause us to drift towards war. For us to live in harmony, it requires that each of us lives in harmony with ourselves."

—Udo Erasmus

PART II

RESOLVING TRAUMA AND BUILDING RESILIENCY

CHAPTER 7

MODERN THERAPIES

At 60, Diane was convinced that all she needed were hormones to fix her brain fog and lack of libido.

She was wrong.

Diane's sister had raved about a new functional medicine practitioner she was seeing who had given her hormone replacements. She was feeling better than ever. Diane wanted what her sister had, so she made an appointment with this new doctor.

During her first appointment, Diane told the doctor that she wanted hormones too. "I want to feel more energized, clear headed, and I want a libido," Diane explained as she kept scratching her arms. Her doctor finally asked if she would roll up her sleeves, and much to her doctor's surprise, both of Diane's arms were covered in hives.

"I get them every time I travel, and I just got back from the East Coast visiting my granddaughter," Diane told her doctor. "This has been going on about twenty-five years, maybe longer. I usually have to go on prednisone, which my general practitioner prescribes. It's the only thing that takes them away."

Diane didn't realize it, but her new functional medicine practitioner was also a trauma-informed psychotherapist. She started asking Diane questions about her childhood using the ACE Test, which asks 10 questions about common adverse childhood experiences of trauma. It turned out that Diane had survived terrible abuse, where

Diane had caught one of her parents having an affair, who told Diane that if she ever told anyone, she'd be killed.

There were so many traumatic moments in Diane's childhood that carried into adulthood that it was manifesting on her skin and in her hormonal imbalance (which was indeed off) and obesity.

It was going to take a lot more than hormones to help Diane resolve her trauma and bring her body and mind back into balance.

OUR TRIALS

What a time to be alive. We are blessed to live during a period when more of us are waking up and wanting to resolve our traumas. We want to stop intergenerational trauma from continuing. We want our children to grow up with different experiences. And we want to live as the best versions of ourselves—happy, healthy, energetic, and loving.

We have therapists and healers who have undertaken their own trauma journeys. They intimately understand and can relate to us. Finally, we have at our fingertips many different therapies and healing modalities that can help us resolve our traumas.

In this chapter, we're exploring the most common and effective therapies that our trauma experts are using to help their patients heal their mind, body, and mind-body levels, including cognitive behavioral therapy, somatic experiencing, EMDR, and body massage.

It's by no means an exhaustive list, and there is no such thing as "the best" or "the number one most effective treatment in the entire world." Asking what's the best therapy is like quizzing 20 people on their favorite food. You will get different answers. What helps you may not help your best friend and vice versa.

Some treatments appear to be more effective for certain traumas. For example, people who have "Big T" traumas seem to do well with therapies like somatic experiencing and EMDR, both of which help your body to release stored pain.

Generally, it takes a healthy dose of curiosity to discover what therapies work for you. If you find something that doesn't jive with you, stay positive. It's not a sign that you'll be hostage to your trauma forever. It means you're one step closer to finding the right fit.

This idea goes for any therapist or healer. You deserve to find the right therapies *and* therapists. Find someone you feel safe with, someone you can trust, someone with whom you will create a safe space to do this deep inner work. Go with your gut. If the therapist feels wrong to you or makes you feel worse about yourself after a session, smash the eject button, stat, and find someone else to work with.

Never feel guilty or bad about leaving with a therapist (or any health practitioner). Dr. Keesha Ewers, an integrative medicine practitioner and psychotherapist, said she tells her patients to imagine shopping for a therapist like they would a pair of shoes. You don't have to buy the first pair you try on.[1]

No matter what therapy you decide to try, make sure you work with a *trauma-informed therapist*. This is someone who has training in trauma-informed care. We cannot underline how critical this is to your recovery and resiliency.

People with this specific training know how to work with trauma, and they have a philosophy that informs their approach. Meaning they create a safe space and trust with their patients so that the patients feel seen, heard, and accepted no matter what.

As you work through this chapter, try to notice your inner response. If a therapy seems interesting, you feel excited, you get shivers, or you just have a sense deep down that something is right, make note. That's your intuition and instinct calling to you—trust it, heed it, and work with it. It will guide you to where and who you need to work with.

And, if you can, try to approach this chapter with some lightness and dare we say, fun(?). Yes, resolving trauma can feel hard, and there's work, commitment, and focus involved, but the outcome is extraordinary. Unresolved trauma is like pulling an 80-pound wagon with you everywhere you go. When you resolve the trauma, you release that wagon, and you will feel lighter. In turn, you'll feel happier, more joyful, and more connected to this world, the people around you, and yourself.

You will *want* to keep going on your road to recovery and beyond with your new therapy or therapist.

May you remain curious and continue to trust your instincts and feel invigorated. You can unwind your trauma. You can feel lighter, more joyful, and peaceful. Let it start right now.

TREATING THE MIND

To resolve trauma, we have to get to the root of it. Anxiety, depression, personality or mood changes, anger, flashbacks, and rage are the results of trauma, not the causes. In some schools of thought, targeting the mind makes the biggest difference. It's considered top-down, working from the head down a little into the body (although the body is not the focus with these therapies).

Therapies focused on the mind can help you uncover any false beliefs and damaging stories that were created about the world, people, and yourself to help deal with the traumas. By identifying and acknowledging the inner tales, you can help rewrite and reframe them. It's a way to process and make sense of what happened while creating a new vision for the world around you.

Many of these therapies have fundamentally changed people's outlook on life and themselves forever. And bonus, many therapies teach tools and techniques you can use outside the therapist's office. Not only do you resolve the previous traumas, you build resiliency to protect you from future experiences too.

Two of the therapies that came up multiple times in our interviews included:

- Cognitive Behavioral Therapy
- Psychoanalytic Therapy

Cognitive Behavioral Therapy

Trauma often rewrites our thoughts, twisting them into negative stories and beliefs we create about ourselves, the world, and people. These negative thoughts lead to negative emotions. Often, we're not even aware of our thoughts or emotions. They just happen. Over time, all of these negative thoughts and emotions impact our body and our spirit, dragging us down, keeping us in pain, and making life feel dark.

Cognitive behavioral therapy (CBT) is a talk therapy that gets at the negative thoughts around our trauma and the stories and beliefs we create from them. If we can change the story and the words we use, then we can change our lives.

How powerful are words? Try this. Close your eyes and say no, ten times. Notice how your chest, arms, legs, stomach, and entire body feel when you say that word.

Now close your eyes again and say yes ten times. Notice the difference?

When we say no, our body involuntarily tenses. When we say yes, it relaxes, and we soften and gently open.

This is part of what CBT teaches. It shows you how to notice the negative script that's constantly playing in the background of your life and then flip it to something positive. Dr. Carl Totton, a clinical psychologist, uses a practice called snap, stop, notice, and pause. "If you can stop that negative path of thinking, notice it, and then you can begin to rewrite the script," Dr. Totton explained.[2] "You can change the narrative. You can do positive reframes from cognitive behavioral therapy."[3]

Dr. Totton said if we can just catch ourselves as soon as we think or feel bad, it can go a long way toward creating a new experience of life and rewriting the trauma script that got written.

CBT is used to help treat many ailments, including PTSD, anxiety, depression, eating disorders, grief, and chronic illness. We should note that if you have suffered a "Big T" trauma and you have a strong terror or fear physiological response that's stored in your body, by itself, CBT probably won't get you all the way to releasing that pain. CBT is great to move you out of the negative thinking and self-talk, but you'll need something to help your body let go—just telling it to, unfortunately, won't work.

If you're interested in CBT, you may also want to check out a body-based therapy or start with one of the mind-body treatments such as EMDR.

Psychoanalytic Therapy

Do "Little t" traumas haunt you? If so, then you may want to consider psychoanalytic psychotherapy. Therapists trained in this practice will sit with their clients and feel from them what kinds of developmental and potential early traumas they have experienced that have shaped their view of themselves, others, and the world.

According to psychologist Dr. Sam Rader, psychoanalysis tries to address the first five years of life, not by analyzing with our brains but by allowing us to have a new experience of those formative years using the therapist as a stand-in for "good enough" caregivers.

"The ways [clients] engage with the world is a reflection of their early experience, then they bring that way of engaging into the room with [therapists]," explained Dr. Rader. "That's what we call transference, and even though it can be quite painful for them to project their early material onto us, it's a wonderful opportunity for us to slow it down and give the client a new experience."[4]

For example, if you didn't feel heard or seen as a child, then in this therapy setting the therapist will validate, acknowledge, and meet those needs as you had wanted from your parents or primary caregiver. "We give them what they didn't get back, and then reparent them, and they come out of the work less traumatized, more whole, more integrated, and more of who they really are," shared Dr. Rader.[5]

TREATING THE BODY

At the age of 14, William Hufschmidt, a yoga teacher and bodyworker who practices time massage and structural integration (also known as Rolfing), was in a car accident. He barely survived. He had the jaws of life used on him, and he spent six weeks in the hospital recovering from injuries to his leg, which was left shattered and mangled from his ankle up to his groin.

Now in his fifties, he has spent his life healing and giving himself opportunities to grow from his traumatic experience. Yet even today, the repercussions are still vibrant in his body—even if he's not conscious of them.

"I'm doing a lot of work with the scar on the side of my leg, and it brings up an incredible amount of emotion," he shared with us. "I've had memories come up of lying in the hospital bed, of being back in the car, and this is thirty-six years later. Memories are coming up that I haven't even considered before."[6]

William's story is almost identical to Stephanie Speights's, an eco-spiritual practitioner. During a lymphatic massage, as soon as the massage therapist started working on her upper thigh and hips, Stephanie started weeping as a memory of her father came into her mind. Six months ago, her father had died in a tragic accident. "I was so busy with busy-ness that I didn't have time to grieve," she said to us. "I'm positive I was holding the grief in my thighs and hips, and when [the massage therapist] started working on that spot, the grief just poured out of me."[7]

Stephanie tried to stop the pain, but she couldn't. She felt a little embarrassed, but her massage therapist told her not to worry and that it was common with her patients.

This is the story of bodywork and trauma, and it's also why making this pit stop on your journey is worthwhile. Not only do these therapies just feel good, they can reach spots where we've stored trauma that we don't even realize we have.

Bodywork is a way to reconnect with your body. The road to recovery is learning how to be at home in our physical selves, to feel and notice what our body's saying, and to be aligned with it. Bodywork can be a gentle walk back to your physical self, creating greater awareness and connection for you. "We can talk about bodywork as an opportunity," said William. "Instead of me doing something to my client, my intention is to summon them to that place in their body that my hands are. I'm bringing their awareness to the tissue."[8]

For some of us, feeling pleasure is hard. We may have come from a strict religious upbringing that taught us feeling good was bad, or we may have been physically harmed. Bodywork can then help retrain our bodies and minds that touch, physical sensation, and pleasure are actually okay.

Bodywork comes in many forms and often with specialties and subcategories. Some of the more common bodywork therapies the experts we spoke with continually mentioned included:

- Massage therapy (Deep Tissue, Shiatsu, Swedish, Reflexology)
- Myofascial release
- Craniosacral release
- Chiropractic
- Acupressure or acupuncture
- Reiki
- Rolfing (combines myofascial release with movement)
- Floatation (when you're floating in a saltwater bath in a deep tank, in sensory deprivation with no sound and darkness, and all you do is focus on your breath and relaxing)

Because of the hands-on nature of this therapy, it's even more important that you find someone you can trust, relax, and feel safe with. Sometimes this may take a few sessions as both you and your bodyworker get used to each other.

For many people, regular bodywork plays a big part in their resiliency practices. Some people will go once a month to their chiropractor or massage therapist for tune-ups, but how often you use bodywork depends on your unique journey. If you can, try to explore different therapies. See what feels right to your body, and remember that what you may use today can change in five years or it could be in your life forever.

There's no right or wrong here—there's only what's right for you.

TREATING THE MIND-BODY CONNECTION

We can work with our minds. We can work with our bodies. And we can work with our minds *and* bodies simultaneously. That's the idea behind the therapies that focus on helping the body release trauma while rewiring the brain. Common therapies that treat the mind-body connection are:

- Somatic therapy
- Eye movement desensitization reprocessing (EMDR)

- Emotional freedom technique (also known as tapping)
- Art, music, or dance therapy

Let's dive deeper into them.

Somatic Therapy

Your body stores trauma, and while it would be nice if we could just tell it to "let go," it usually takes a little more prodding. Enter somatic therapies, which focus on helping your nervous system to release the trauma it's stored from the mind and body.

We experience trauma as a very intense visceral sensation in our bodies. Somatic experience is about sensing the places in the body where an activation takes place, whether it's from tightness, tension, too much or too little energy, or where something feels stuck.

"The beautiful thing about the human mind and body is that it's so resilient and so self-healing, all you do in somatic experiencing is sit with a client and have them sense into their bodies and into these sensations associated with trauma," explained Dr. Sam Rader.

"As the client feels the sensation in their body, it's like a mirror for their brain. 'This is the state we're in; this is what we're experiencing.' And then the brain and body right themselves. They start to come back to a healthier baseline. They start to discharge any excess charge and to unwind any excess tension. They start to enliven the places where there was deadness. It just happens naturally. We're connected to our animal selves that know what to do with trauma."[9]

Peter Levine created somatic experiencing by watching wild animals. They are always in danger, yet we never witness a traumatic stress response in them. That's because there's a self-regulating, biological response that helps them release the traumatic experience. When they're in grave danger and their nervous systems go into fight, flight, or freeze, or when the danger has passed and they know they're safe, they will release that burst of energy. They shake, twitch, and convulse that energy out of their body.

Even though we may forget this, we're animals too.

When we're threatened, the same stress hormones will flood our systems. When the threat passes, that tremendous energy outflow has to go somewhere. We usually stop the release. It's too much for us to handle—partly because no one taught us what to do with it. We're biologically damming up the river. When this happens, we stop our nervous system from returning to its rest-and-digest sense of ease and safety.

With somatic experiencing, we track what's going on in the nervous system through the story we tell in our bodies.

When your therapist creates more safety for you, it allows the incomplete fight, flight, or freeze response to be completed.

For some people, finding meaning in and making sense of their trauma is a key part of their resolution. But with somatic experiencing, it's not central. It's about working with the direct, felt, lived experience that you're having in your body, and you don't need to know or remember where your trauma came from.

"The body wants to right itself, to discharge and to come back to homeostasis and baseline," explained Dr. Rader. "Just by feeling into the body allows the brain and body to reorganize and heal."[10]

Somatic experiencing is often used to help people treat "Big T" traumas such as sexual or physical abuse, and PTSD, whether or not they were experienced during childhood or adulthood. It tends to be effective for those who have trauma stuck in the body where the nervous system has been hijacked and is operating in danger mode 24/7.

Eye Movement Desensitization Reprocessing (EMDR)

Remembering "Big T" traumas can be too horrific and retraumatizing for the body and mind to recall. Eye movement desensitization reprocessing (EMDR) takes the traumatic memories stored in the amygdala and helps us reprocess them so they no longer trigger an intense fear response or PTSD symptoms. EMDR works on a wide range of "Big T" and "Little t" traumas. A trained therapist will stand in front of you, hold up a finger, and ask you to track their side-to-side motion with your eyes. This movement lights up the right and left parts of your brain. Simultaneously, the therapist may also snap in your ears for an auditory stimulation or alternately tap on acupressure points on your body.

You will start by calling up the traumatic memory, going to the worst part of the moment. You speak to what you remember, and as you do this, the therapist moves their finger in front of your eyes and you follow it side to side. At some point, the therapist will pause you so you can take a deep breath and then slowly exhale before moving on to the next stage.

"The technique doesn't require any intervention from the therapist," explained Dr. Sam Rader. "We don't give any interpretations. We don't try to move the process along in any way, so the client's internal healing resources show up. As soon as they start reprocessing this trauma, it becomes integrated very naturally."[11]

If the memories become too painful, the therapist will remind you that you're in the here and now while continuing to do the side-to-side eye movement. As the memories dislodge, the therapist reminds you that no matter what you're remembering, you will be okay. They're helping you to awaken a different connection in your body and mind to the memory, so instead of feeling intense fear and fright, you begin to look at the trauma from a distance as something that happened. Through this process, you may see what the trauma has taught you and the people who may have shown up to help you along this journey.

Thought Field Therapy/Emotional Freedom Technique/Tapping

When you were growing up, did someone teach you how to engage your nervous system? Did they show you how to take a difficult experience and move it through your mind and body?

If you're like most people, it's an emphatic no. But you can learn to instantly release the trapped energy and difficult emotions stored in your mind and body simply by tapping on acupressure points on your body.

This is what Dr. Carl Totton used to help a student who was struggling to process and integrate an intense experience. Dr. Totton was working as a psychologist in a high school when one morning, a 16-year-old boy was sent to see him. The teenager had been sitting in the back of his English class, hyperventilating, shaking, and sobbing hysterically.

"I had never seen this boy; there were like 2,500 kids in the high school," Dr. Totton recalled.[12] "I tried to get a little history. He told me over the weekend he was working as a box boy in a supermarket. They got robbed, and someone put a gun to his head. Freaked him out. Probably would have freaked me out too. I don't blame him, but he's having a full panic attack, and I'm thinking, *If I don't do something quickly, these symptoms that he's having right now are going to get embedded in his body, mind, and cellular structure, leaving him vulnerable to being triggered by things that remind him of the experience for the rest of his life.*"[13]

Dr. Totton used one of the most powerful tools he knew: tapping. He had studied under Dr. Roger Callahan, the clinical psychologist who founded tapping, which combines ancient Chinese medicine acupuncture points with modern psychology. "If you just tap on some of those points that are for physical healing, they also accomplish emotional healing," explained Dr. Totton.

For about 10 minutes, Dr. Totton had the teen tap on certain acupuncture points. As the boy did, his breathing became calmer. He stopped crying, hysterically shaking, and feeling out of control.

When they started the tapping, he had asked the boy on a scale of 1 to 10, with 10 being the worst you can imagine, how he felt. Unsurprisingly, the boy said he was a 10. After about four minutes of tapping, Dr. Totton asked him again how he felt. The boy started smiling and said a 4, maybe a 5, so Dr. Totton had him keep tapping. After another five minutes, the teen started laughing, saying he was a 1, maybe a 2, so Dr. Totton told him to keep going but this time added some EMDR. The teen now was tapping and following Dr. Totton's finger for about 30 seconds.

Finally, the teen said he was back to 0. From start to finish it took 20 minutes, and the teen walked out of Dr. Totton's office smiling.

This happened in real time, but you can use tapping to release any energy and trauma block, no matter how long it's been trapped. Some trainers will also pair tapping with affirmations like "I am safe," "I am strong," "I am calm," or "I am resourceful" to help ease the mind and body to release the trauma that's stored.

Expressive Arts Therapy

Often, it's hard to access our stored pain and release our emotions and thoughts. Sometimes, we don't want to talk about them, and we may not even have the words to describe how we feel or think about our traumas.

Maybe you were a child from a war-torn country and you were forced to leave your home and settle in a foreign nation. Maybe you lived through a devastating natural disaster that decimated your home or village. Maybe as a person of color you've experienced racism at every turn in your life, and you feel the effects of it as it's been passed from generation to generation. Maybe you lost all faith in humanity and God after being abused by a religious leader.

There are so many experiences that feel too big to unwind. Enter *expressive therapies*, which use creative arts to help heal you. You can use these therapies one-on-one with a therapist or in a group community setting, which can relieve feelings of isolation. When we've experienced trauma, we tend to pull away and take ourselves out of personal interactions and connections. It's understandable. We may feel ashamed or scared to be vulnerable with others. Our experiences may have taught us that people are dangerous and we shouldn't trust them—and rightfully so, some people are. But there are also many safe, caring, and supportive people who understand you and who want to help support you, just as you probably want to support them too.

The focus is more on the process of creating and what you're experiencing while it happens and less on the final result.

We're going to take a brief peek into the three most common expressive art therapies. If you're interested in exploring an expressive art therapy form, then look for someone who is trained and board-certified.

Art Therapy

"Art is something that is beyond our emotions, beyond our mind, even beyond anything other than our spirit," Dr. Lin Morel, a spiritual advisor and life coach, told us.[14] For 20 years, she has worked with a nonprofit specializing in helping people who have survived domestic violence and veterans who have been impacted by "Big T" traumas. She estimates that she's worked with at least 400,000 people who have all benefited from doing art therapy.

"Art bypasses all our defenses," she said. "Most people are not an artist, and it's not about being an artist. It's about letting you express yourself."[15]

Dr. Morel believes that art therapy is especially helpful for people who experienced significant trauma in childhood. As children, we don't have the words to describe what's happened to us on an emotional level. But you can draw, paint, create a collage, or sculpt the feeling.

Sometimes, Dr. Morel will prompt people to draw specific images like a monster or, alternately, what is safe to them. Other times, she'll have them scribble on paper using whatever colors they want. Sometimes she has them decorate suitcases to reflect what they are running from or toward. When a patient is dealing with fear, anger, or violent thoughts and feelings, she'll have them blow up a bunch of balloons and then pop them, as if they're popping their pain and big emotions.

When you're engaged in art therapy, you can also get the benefits of meditation. You're constantly being brought into the present moment. You have to choose what color, shape, line, collage materials, or piece of clay to use.

"The art process can bring information forward that may not be as accessible through other modalities," explained Darcy Lubbers, a psychotherapist, board-certified clinical art therapist, and somatic psychotherapist.[16] "It brings forward information that people maybe had suppressed for a very long time and weren't in touch with, or never felt there was a safe space to express them. When you do the artwork, it just spills out onto the page, and you get a chance to look at it and notice things that you weren't aware of, and that can be very healing."[17]

Music Therapy

"The beautiful thing about music therapy is it's a container for people who may feel afraid to express their emotions that would otherwise come out in a destructive manner or get pushed down and would come out as depression or another issue," explained Stacie Aamon Yeldell, a board-certified music psychotherapist.[18]

If you're resistant to talk therapies or psychoanalysis, music therapy could be a powerful alternative. Music is faster than words. It bypasses the ego and goes right to your heart, so the feeling and emotion that you have stored immediately gets released. Think about when you listen to the radio and a song comes on that reminds you of your ex. You feel something instantly whether you want to or not. This is what can happen with music therapy.

"The ego is always just trying to protect us," explained Stacie. "The ego doesn't know the difference between transformation and annihilation, so anytime we're trying to change, evolve, or grow, the ego is like, 'Oh my God, I'm going to die. I think that she's trying to kill me. Nope.' When we encounter resistance in therapy or change, it's your ego trying to protect you and keep you locked in the status quo. Music helps to bypass all that, get you to your feeling state, and then once you start to feel, all the doors open. You begin to experience whatever it is that needs to be experienced, like the trauma from before, and you are having that experience within the safe container again."[19]

In one of Stacie's group therapy programs, she used songwriting and music to help girls who had been sexually abused at camp to release their emotions and integrate the trauma. Stacie chose a theme each session, such as shame. Then every girl shared what she felt about it like "I feel ashamed when this happened to me . . ." or "I feel like no one will ever look at me the same."

Everyone has a chance to share on this theme, and their words get used in a song. "It wasn't just songwriting, it was therapy group," Stacie told us. By the end, the group took what emerged from their discussions and created a song with verses and a chorus.

Once the song was written, Stacie would play either the piano or guitar while asking the girls what the song felt like—was it up-tempo, melancholy, or both? Once they picked the vibe, Stacie played a few chords and the improvisation began. Some girls sang and others who may have felt shy played a shaker or rattle, but everyone had a chance to be a part of the song. "Everyone participated in the expression of this beautiful thing that they've created, which is holding the experience of the group. Music is a container. The song they wrote is a collaboration of all their shared experiences. All their pain is being held in that song, then alchemized into something beautiful that feels good and is absolutely healing to be able to express that," Stacie said.[20]

Dance Therapy

Dance movement therapy is the idea that your mind and body aren't separate. Everything you have experienced in your life, you have experienced in your body—including every good moment, every trauma, every sadness, every rite of passage. The theory behind dance therapy is that if you're trying to deal with your emotions, only working with the memories in your mind isn't enough, because your body holds them too.

Dance therapy is a way to look at what you're going through in life and to move through it. Gabrielle Kaufman, a therapist who specializes in perinatal mental health and trauma, uses dance therapy with her clients. How it works is she'll ask a client how they feel and then talk them through releasing it. For example, if someone says, "I feel like I have the weight of the world on me. I'm so overwhelmed. I feel like I'm carrying a boulder on my back," then she asks them to move as if that boulder is on their back.

As they're moving, she keeps asking questions and guiding them into the feeling of their bodies. "Feel the muscle tension in your body," she may say, or "Feel that crouching or that constriction of breathing. What is causing that? What does that remind you of? Are there stories related to it?"

As we move our bodies, we recall stories from our past. We're recalling that stored trauma and memory. This is not easy! Many people reach a certain point of "No more! Get me off this ride!"

This is the fork in the road. They can choose to do something with that boulder. Gabrielle may ask, "Do you want to take it off?" Sometimes they say no, but they may want a little help holding it, so Gabrielle will help lift it a bit, asking them, "How does it feel now? What do you want to do next?"

"It's giving them that sense of autonomy and this idea that they have a part in their own healing, especially the healing for stories that they just held on to deeply in their body," Gabrielle explained. "Movement is just this beautiful experience to really release."[21]

Gabrielle shared a story of working with "Karey," a woman who had been sexually molested multiple times. For Karey, her body and skin had become this painful place to live and experience the world in. Working with Gabrielle, Karey imagined herself as a snake and moved like the reptile. As she kept moving, the image of shedding her skin slowly came into her mind. Together, Karey and Gabrielle explored that experience.

Gabrielle would ask, "What would it be like if you could shed your skin? What would it be like to take control and go through that painful experience? What does it feel like to let go of that skin? How does that open you up for more moving? How does this open you for making new choices or for creating a new skin that's of your choosing?"

Through this process, Karey began making sense of her traumas. She felt that shedding her skin and growing a fresh, new one was painful. Yet she kept seeing the image of a new skin forming. "What comes forward often are intuitive healing pictures," Gabrielle explained.[22]

You just need permission and space, gentleness, and patience with yourself to work through the process.

THE ROAD TO RECOVERY

Diane's doctor took a multiprong approach to help her heal. First, she ran Diane through a battery of tests to find out if she had any food sensitivities, hormone imbalances, adrenal deficiencies, or imbalances in her microbiome.

The tests revealed Diane had an overgrowth of bacteria, which was treated immediately. Next, was diet. Diane went on an anti-inflammatory plan that removed dairy, alcohol, sugar, and processed carbs from her diet. She began walking outdoors for at least 20 minutes every day, and she was on a strict bedtime routine—no screens for at least an hour before bed and lights out by 10 P.M.

The last puzzle piece came from EMDR. Treating the underlying traumas would be the only way to help Diane's mind and body return to balance. It would also help her low libido and brain fog. Diane was willing to try anything and she trusted her doctor, so once a week for 50 minutes, Diane had an EMDR treatment.

Within six weeks, she had lost 15 pounds of water weight and bloating as the inflammation in her body went down. She had more energy, wanted to have sex with her husband, and for the first time in her life, she felt real joy. Even more amazing for her, the hives disappeared—without ever having to pop a steroid pill.

About a year after she had completed her therapy, Diane was still doing great. She texted her doctor a picture of herself doing a yoga pose as she visited her granddaughter on the East Coast.

Diane had a new life and had met a version of herself that she never knew had existed.

Then just three months later, she broke out in hives all over her legs. She went back to her doctor to figure out what had gone sideways. It wasn't her diet or exercise. She was still keeping up with that. But she had a huge emotional eruption during a family reunion, and it retriggered a lot of her old traumas.

Diane did another round of EMDR, and she talked to her doctor about other therapies, treatments, and self-nurturing practices that could help her on her road to recovery. Diane went on to try somatic experiencing, meditating, and breathwork, and she went on two yoga retreats every year to help keep the hives at bay. She also learned that when she interacted with difficult family members, she needed to double-down on self-care before and after the interaction.

Diane still had her peaks and valleys. There were (and still are) challenging times that hit old scripts, patterns, and traumas. But she knows she has the inner resources and the external support to help see her through, and she's become more attuned to her body and its signals so that she knows when she needs to return to a therapy.

This is the true road to recovery. Releasing trauma often happens in waves. Accepting where we are in each moment and finding the trusted allies and resources is the secret. Diane discovered the modern therapies that worked best for her, and that's all any of us can do. EMDR may be the right choice for you now, or maybe it's cognitive thought therapy. Two years from now, this may change, and that's okay. Patience and persistence, paired with greater inner awareness, have helped Diane slowly release her trauma and reengage with her life on healthier and happier terms. This awaits you too.

REFLECTIONS

Were you drawn to any modern therapies? Did any of them seem interesting? It can be helpful to start by exploring therapies that intrigue you or that seem like they could be a good fit. Conversely, if you've walked your road to recovery for some time, then perhaps it's time to try a new approach. Were there any that you haven't attempted? Aim to identify at least one modern therapy that you want to learn more about. That doesn't mean you will go full-throttle on it—unless you feel all in, and if that's the case, go for it. Researching to explore more about a modern therapy can be a powerful next step in this journey. From there, you can learn what practitioners may be working in your area. Bonus: if you identified the source for your trauma in Part I, then see if you can match effective treatments by using this chapter as a guide.

SAGE WISDOM

"We can choose to see trauma either as empowering or disempowering. The meaning we make of it, the perspective we bring, will either be life giving or life draining. No matter what the trauma has been, no matter how difficult or how long it's been there, with some support we have the ability in us to transform our experience, not of what happened, but of future life."

—Mary Morrissey

CHAPTER 8

ANCIENT TRADITIONS AND NATURAL REMEDIES

As a sergeant first class Special Forces Green Beret, Andrew had been in life-and-death situations during multiple deployments. There was never a problem—until his last one. That's when the extreme fatigue, loss of libido, behavioral issues, and deep, dark depression began.

It made no sense to him. He loved his life. Andrew had always wanted to be a special forces operator. As a top performer, he was at the tip of the spear, part of a small, elite group. On the home front, he was married to the woman of his dreams, and they had five children (today it's seven).

Andrew was living his dream life. Still, every morning he woke up feeling not just a little down, but like his family had been murdered. He knew it was bad, so he reached out to the military medical system, and they immediately put him in psychotherapy and prescribed him medication.

It didn't help. If anything, it made Andrew's symptoms worse. He started experiencing anxiety and panic attacks. He struggled with speech and other cognitive functioning, and then the physiological problems began, including losing his balance. Doctors diagnosed him with new psychological conditions. They told him that he had seen so much combat that his mind had compartmentalized all of these operations—but there were too many for his mind to contain. His mind's filing cabinet couldn't close, and everything was spilling out.

Andrew understood the rationale and acknowledged that for some people that's likely the case. But he didn't feel he was one of them. He wasn't hung up on any experiences. Nothing haunted him, and he wasn't having flashbacks. The diagnosis didn't feel right, but what did he know?

The doctors also told him that he had suffered a number of traumatic brain injuries. Part of Andrew's work was to set up explosives. In his ten years, he had been knocked unconscious only once, but he had been present for thousands of explosions.

An injured brain? What does that mean? Andrew wondered. The doctors didn't have many answers, but they put him on more medication. They didn't work either. Andrew continued to deteriorate.

Forced to medically retire, Andrew's dream life had twisted into a nightmare. He started drinking heavily. He wasn't sleeping or eating well. His doctors told him that his wife would have to take care of him for the rest of his life. They advised him to bring a pen and paper wherever he went—that's how bad his memory was. Some days, he couldn't remember how to drive home.

Then there was the uncontrollable, spontaneous rage. Normal interactions would quickly turn into arguments or physical fights. He would get so wound up that he would go upstairs and lock himself in his bedroom closet. He'd lay in the fetal position, sometimes for hours, until the energy and rage had subsided.

One day, he was yelling at one of his kids, but he didn't remember what was going on. When he came to, all he saw was the horrified look on his child's face.

A number of guys in his special force's community had died by suicide, and Andrew had never understood why on earth these tried-and-true warriors would ever choose that path. Now he could. For the first time ever, Andrew thought that maybe life would be better for his family if he removed himself from the equation forever.

One night, he almost did. He stopped just in the nick of time, realizing how much more pain and harm he would cause to his wife and children. He couldn't do that to them, but he also couldn't keep living like this. He needed help different from what he was receiving, but what and where would he find it?

OUR TRIALS

We live in a culture of trauma.

It's always humming in the background, but most people are moving too fast to see it. Keep going. Never stop. Be more productive and efficient. Make more money. Achieve more success. Look a certain way. Buy more stuff. Shove more "doing" into our days.

In this hurried and harried culture, we've lost our connection between our inner and outer worlds. As humans, we live in both. Unresolved trauma closes us off from the internal experience of noticing what's happening inside our bodies, minds, hearts, and souls. Our inner world is our compass for navigating the external physical reality. Without it, more of our lived experiences become traumatic.

Culturally, we don't like to talk about this, but if we're being honest and staring reality in the face, the truth of life is that it can, and often does, bring heartache, struggle, and pain. The people we love die, sometimes much sooner than we want. Serious illnesses, natural disasters, and terrible accidents that are random and seemingly meaningless happen. Sometimes we're betrayed by spouses, lovers, and friends. Sometimes as kids, we don't get what we need from our parents or caregivers, and as adults we lose jobs, homes, marriages, and children. Dreams get crushed as we fail and fall. We suffer losses and disappointments.

And life is beautiful too.

Opportunities arise that we could never have planned. We meet people in the most serendipitous of ways, and they become our best friends. We meet and fall in love. Maybe we get married. Maybe we have kids and grandkids who open our minds and hearts to seeing how amazing this world truly is. Maybe we travel and see the world. We learn about ourselves through hobbies and interests. We read books, watch movies or plays or television shows, we listen to the radio or a podcast, we take in art, and we're stunned by the new ideas and the beauty that comes from these acts of creation.

Through it all, we laugh and cry because life is about the good and the bad, the happy and the sad, the triumphs and the defeats.

Life. It's messy and unpredictable, and oh, so beautiful and wonderful and worth experiencing every breath.

The spectrum of life—the heartaches and the heart openings—has always been the human experience.

Every human being throughout history has wrestled with these universal struggles and faced traumatic moments. No one goes through this world unscathed. Today, trauma and turmoil constantly bombard us. From terrifying news headlines to social media feeds to our entertainment, sometimes it can feel like trauma stalks us everywhere.

One of the biggest differences between the past and present is that today, most of us have no guideposts teaching us *how* to move through challenging experiences or what remedies to use when events leave us in deep, inner pain and turmoil. Without this resiliency, we walk around wounded and devastated by trauma that we may, or may not, recognize.

However, turn history's pages and you'll find lessons for how to recover and build inner strength and resiliency. For thousands of years, indigenous and ancient people used their diets and movement to heal. The ancient wise ones regularly turned to Mother Nature for help, and they performed sacred healing rituals and ceremonies to restore balance in the body, mind, heart, and soul and to reconnect their inner and outer worlds.

Thankfully, much of this wisdom still exists.

Trauma experts are using ancient wisdom and natural remedies to help release our blocks from trauma, and some are merging technology of today with solutions of the past to create new treatments and protocols. This is what we're exploring in this chapter. We'll look at some of the most effective tools for restoring your biochemistry, tweaking your diet, adding more movement and exercise into your day, meditating, spending time in Mother Nature, using plant medicine, and performing sacred rituals and ceremonies.

As you move through this stop on our trauma journey, think of each option as a *possible* complement to some of the therapies we discussed earlier *and* as part of a resiliency kit you're building. If one or two practices really jump out at you, find out more information. Look for experts in your area whom you can work with, or talk with your therapist about adding some of these tools to your plan.

Open yourself to new possibilities. And keep in mind, if you try one treatment—whether it's one method or another—and it doesn't work, that's okay. Try another, and then another, and keep going until you find those that work for *you*.

Keep asking the questions and seeking the answers. Never allow someone to tell you it's hopeless or your trauma is too deep to resolve. Just as life can be hard and painful, it can also be sweet and filled with pleasure. Let your will to recover and your determination to reach the other side of this fortify your spirit and guide you forward.

BALANCING YOUR BIOCHEMISTRY

"When you've had childhood trauma or when you constantly feel overwhelmed because you're exposed to trauma on a daily basis, the biochemistry of the body shifts," Dr. Keesha Ewers, an integrative medicine practitioner and trauma-informed psychotherapist, told us.[1]

If you're exhausted all the time, feel depressed or anxious, have no to low sex drive, and have the sense that your body feels off, then you may have very real chemical imbalances that need addressing. Dr. Ewers uses a multiprong approach to treating her patients, running full biomarkers, testing their microbiomes for any imbalances, looking into food sensitivities, and checking for vitamin, mineral, and hormone deficiencies, and exposure to toxins.

Simultaneously, Dr. Ewers will treat her patients' physiology, and she'll address any underlying traumas using trauma-informed, psychotherapeutic approaches like EMDR or psychotherapy.

Dr. Mark L. Gordon, a neuroendocrinologist who specializes in TBIs, addresses the hormones of the brain and body using mostly natural remedies. "Eighty to ninety percent of what we use are naturopathic products," he said.[2]

Using a personalized protocol, patients may receive treatments that include supplements, hormone replacement, probiotics, and new dietary guidelines. Many of his patients report incredible results. For instance, he worked with a captain in the air force who was seeing a psychiatrist and a speech therapist because she had lost her speaking ability. Within six weeks of treatment, both the psychiatrist and speech therapist said they weren't needed. Dr. Gordon has helped wheelchair-dependent veterans regain the ability to walk, and he's helped people get off dozens of prescription medications.

Trauma can affect us in strange ways that we'd never imagine. The good news is that you have more options than a prescription from modern Western medicine. This isn't to knock these doctors or that kind of treatment. There is a place and time for everything, and depending on your unique situation, prescriptions may be needed. But on your road to recovery, it may be worth a stop at an integrative or functional medicine practitioner's office, or a trauma-informed therapist who can also test for and understands the biochemistry of your body. Consult and work with your doctor on this. Who knows? One of the keys to unlocking your trauma door may be solving for your unique biochemistry.

FINE-TUNING YOUR DIET AND NUTRITION

Food fuels us, and it can heal us too.

Created thousands of years ago, traditional Chinese medicine and Ayurvedic medicine use what we eat to help restore, and keep, the body, mind, and spirit balanced. When we're balanced, we're healthy.

The challenge in our modern world is that much of the food we eat is harmful and causes a lot of inflammation in the body. Trauma and inflammation are often linked, and the only way you reduce the physiological swelling is by changing your diet.

You'll still need to address unresolved issues, but eliminating some foods while increasing others can make a huge difference in your state of mind and overall well-being.

If you can, work with an integrative or functional medicine practitioner who can run panels and test for vitamin or mineral deficiencies.

They will usually identify what supplements you may need, and doses, and they'll monitor for effectiveness. That's powerful information for anyone with or without trauma.

And there are some tweaks you can likely make now, like adopting an anti-inflammatory diet. You'll eat a lot of fruits like cherries and berries; vegetables such as kale, cabbage, spinach, and broccoli; whole grains including oatmeal, brown rice, and other unrefined grains; plant-based proteins like beans and nuts; herbs such as turmeric and garlic; and fish that have omega-3 fatty acids like tuna and salmon.

You'll cut out stuff everyone loves to eat, but that our bodies don't digest well, including processed foods, sugar, anything fatty or greasy, red meat like beef, dairy like cheese and milk, anything with trans fat (labeled as partially hydrogenated oils), and gluten.

Also, take out alcohol, which ignites inflammation in the brain. It's been found to decrease the production of growth hormone, which Dr. Gordon calls "the ultimate hormone in the body."[3]

If you can, try to eliminate these foods for 30 days. If that's too much right now, then try a week or two and notice how you feel. Keep a journal and track what you notice in your body after a meal. Does your stomach grumble? Do you sprint to the bathroom? Do you feel indigestion or cramps?

If you can, try to eat organic. You'll ingest fewer pesticides, enjoy a small to moderate increase in nutrients, and lower levels of toxic metals like cadmium.[4]

Our bodies speak to us all the time. We just have to relearn how to listen and interpret what they're saying, and doing this through food can be one of the easiest and most beneficial practices.

THE POWER OF MOVEMENT

Movement heals.

That's something the ancients knew thousands of years ago. Yoga, the sister science of Ayurveda, and tai chi and qigong, the sister sciences to traditional Chinese medicine, were developed to help people move energy through the channels of their bodies and organs. The ancients believed (and it's still the theory today) that when energy gets stuck, disease happens.

Trauma is stuck energy. It's why bodywork is so effective. When we move energy through our bodies, we keep our channels clear for future experiences to move through more easily.

Tai chi and qigong are gentle, flowing movements. In qigong, you mix meditation and self-massage to clear the energy channels. Yoga can take many forms; some practices are more vigorous, while others, gentle. There's even such a thing as trauma-informed yoga.

As an added bonus, these practices can bring the mind and body back into harmony, helping you reconnect to your inner life. Practicing yoga, tai chi, or qigong can help you learn the language of your body. Do you notice how a posture or movement makes your muscles feel tight or relaxed? Do you feel them stretching? Are there knots or sharp pains? Do they ache or feel sore? Do you feel strong? Are the movements easy or hard?

The more you practice, the more a reawakening and remembering of your body and mind connection happens. You not only strengthen your muscles, but your mind too with these forms.

Are tai chi, qigong, and yoga the only practices you should attempt? Not necessarily. These three are often cited for their effectiveness and ease in which anyone, at any fitness level and age, can start. But if you've always dreamed of taking a dance or cycling class or wanted to try martial arts, then go for it.

Just make sure you meet your body where it's at. If you haven't been active for a while, take it easy. Build up muscle, stamina, agility, and flexibility slowly.

MOTHER NATURE HEALS

Human beings are a part of nature. We know that's easy to forget in our modern, industrial, technology-driven world—but it's the truth.

Humans are animals. Our ancestors lived with this knowledge. We created our lives with the land, not just on it. We turned to Mother Nature for wisdom, healing, and strength.

We are meant to be in nature, to experience and witness, and to let it heal our trauma wounds. In a UC Berkeley study, researchers found that one week after veterans and at-risk, inner-city youth who experience PTSD symptoms spent a week white-water rafting, on average participants reported a 29 percent reduction in their PTSD symptoms, a 21 percent decrease in general stress, a 10 percent improvement in social relationships, a 9 percent improvement in life satisfaction, and an 8 percent increase in happiness.[5]

Trauma can make us shut down. The pain of our past experiences is just too much to bear, and so we close off our inner selves. But when we disconnect from the pain (as understandable as it is), we also lose the ability to feel the richness of life.

To feel gratitude and awe for the majesty of Mother Nature and the Earth we call home means opening ourselves to feeling pain and heartache from the past. And therein lies our paths to recovery.

When we turn to nature, walking consciously through her, paying attention to all the little details, we remind our inner selves that there's something much bigger than our traumas, bigger than even ourselves. Being with Mother Nature allows us to let small trickles of light into our worlds.

Even if it's just for a moment, that's all it takes. Once you allow a little awe, wonder, and amazement into your life, it grows even brighter. If you spend time outside, preferably away from traffic, noise, and concrete, you will find a gradual reawakening with yourself and the world around you.

Mother Nature can help relieve stress, anxiety, and fear and help your body and mind move from the constant vigilance of danger into a more relaxed space. The more time in nature, the better, but just 20 minutes will do. Research found that 64 percent of participants reported improvement in life satisfaction by spending just 20.5 minutes a day in a park.[6]

Healing from Mother Nature is ancient wisdom that all indigenous people have known and practiced throughout time.

Dr. Carl Totton explained it this way: "All the indigenous medicine men and women around the world, all the shamans, one hundred percent of people that I've studied with, before they do any healing, whether it's mental, emotional, spiritual, or physical, they align themselves to the earth, to nature. They will turn to the south, and they'll say a prayer or blessing, then they'll turn to the west and the north and the east. They'll get down on their hands and knees. They'll touch the earth, look up at the sky. They have aligned themselves emotionally, energetically, spiritually with the protective factors of the earth herself. There's nothing more powerful than that."[7]

If you only try one remedy, make it this one. It costs nothing but gives you so much. Just going outside and sitting under a tree or on a rock, or lying in the grass and taking slow, deep breaths, or walking barefoot and feeling the earth will awaken a deep emotional and energetic healing within you. These practices will slow your nervous system, cleansing you of pain and negativity. This is not something you can ever receive from a gadget or inside a steel building.

Mother Nature heals, but we have to let her in.

MEDITATION

At his psychotherapy practice, Dr. Carl Totton takes an integrative approach with every patient, customizing and individualizing their treatments and the daily techniques and tools he recommends.

But there is one practice that he teaches to every patient: meditation.

Dr. Totton believes that when you have trauma tucked inside, you can't just stop your mind from chattering and make it go blank. It often takes training and time to first learn how to relax, and then to go inward to notice your thoughts and emotions, and then finally to be able to let them go.

How often do you feel triggered by intense anger? Rage? Fear? Impatience? Frustration? Unresolved trauma shortens our fuse, leaving us one comment, act, or thought away from losing our center and melting down. This is largely because our nervous system is so dysregulated that we cannot stay aligned with our inner peace. We're stressed out all the time.

Cue meditation. Throughout the world and for thousands of years, people have used this practice to calm their nervous system, quiet their mind, and lengthen their fuse. As Dr. Mark L. Gordon explained, it also helps balance our biochemistry. "Meditation helps drop cortisol, which drops inflammatory cytokines, which reduces inflammation, which improves our sense of well-being."[8]

We often think of meditation as sitting cross-legged on a cushion on the floor and quieting our minds. This passive meditation aims to make the mind a still pond, without any ripples of thought or emotion.

Instead of teaching passive meditation to his clients, Dr. Totton uses active meditation, or guided imagery. Many of the experts we spoke to use this kind of meditation for their patients as well. With guided imagery, you go *with* your thoughts and any images that arise. Instead of reliving the experience, you watch it as if it's a movie and narrate to your therapist what you see, what's happening, where you are, who you're with, and what you're doing.

Becoming the observer and seeing yourself and your emotions, thoughts, and experiences from a higher vantage point allows you to disconnect some of the intense, emotional charge around your trauma.

Everyone can benefit from meditation, especially people who experienced childhood developmental traumas where our parents couldn't read or understand what we needed at that moment. Through guided meditation, we can go into our memory vault and repair what was broken.

We can use our mind's eye to visualize ourselves asking for and receiving the care that we needed. We become our saviors giving to ourselves what our caregivers couldn't—for whatever reason that may have been.

Most of the experts we spoke with noted the benefits of meditating, and most teach their patients first how to relax, and then to meditate. But they also had a couple of cautionary flags.

First, sometimes we can use meditation (or any spiritual practice) to bypass the trauma in our bodies. You can experience incredible awakenings, *but* if you have trauma stored in your body, it still needs releasing. Especially if you're wrestling with a "Big T" event, which tends to embed in the nervous system.

If you're experiencing PTSD or working through an extreme event such as being in a war zone or car accident, being repeatedly abused as a child, or being assaulted or in a natural disaster, you may want to consider using meditation under the care of a trained therapist or professional. There's a chance meditation could make your trauma symptoms worse or retraumatize you.

In Dr. Totton's practice, if a patient is rewatching an intense experience, Dr. Totton may say, "Okay, put that event on the floor. Now I want you to imagine yourself getting taller all the way up to the clouds. Put your head in the clouds, so your shoulders expand from horizon to horizon. You're putting your feet all the way down to the center of the earth. Now from up there, and as big as you are now, look down at that traumatic event that happened. How does it look? Really small?"

Through this exercise, Dr. Totton helps his patients to change their perspective and perception of the event. This can transform how they feel and experience it in the future. Most people need the care and assistance from an objective observer. A professional trauma-informed therapist can take on this role and help us to reframe and reimagine our trauma.

Meditation is an incredible tool that can bring greater health and wellness to your life, and it's a phenomenal way to build resiliency in this world. The last thing we want to do is scare you away. But we do want you to take care of yourself. For some people, getting some extra guidance or coaching from a meditation expert is healthier than going it alone. There's no shame in needing support as you travel back in time.

PLANT MEDICINE

In the Western world, most of us hear the word *psychedelics* and we think parties, drugs, and wild times. But for thousands of years, many indigenous people in South and North America have used consciousness-altering substances like ayahuasca, psilocybin mushrooms, and San Pedro for healing a variety of issues, including trauma.

Shamans (medicine doctors) will administer plants in the form of tea during a ceremony. Once ingested, this plant medicine is believed to pull out and help us purge (through vomiting and urination) the unresolved pain that's lodged inside of us. As we purge out the old, we awaken to a new reality and a different way to view the world, who we are, and everyone and everything in it—including our trauma experience.

Plant medicine can change how we see what happened to us and our present experience of that event.

But in many countries, including the United States, plant medicine is banned. However, psychedelic-assisted therapy is finding its place in the Western world, especially for treating patients suffering from the symptoms of PTSD, which is notoriously difficult to only treat with psychotherapy. Studies suggest 40–60 percent of PTSD patients do not respond adequately to psychotherapy.[9]

Recently, MDMA-assisted psychotherapy has grabbed headlines. Preclinical and clinical studies have found it can increase empathy, prosocial behavior, and trust between the patient and their therapist, and it can act as a catalyst to improving psychotherapy.[10] One study found that 54.2 percent of patients reported no longer meeting the PTSD criteria after two MDMA sessions versus just 22.6 percent of people who did not take it.[11]

Like with most of the treatments we've discussed, you're not going to do it solo and brew your own ayahuasca tea or take some MDMA while sitting in your bedroom. These treatments have to be used under the guidance and supervision of a trained therapist.

Anything that plays with your consciousness and can move you into different states can help the healing process, but it can also harm you too. Just like in meditation, you want to work with a trusted guide who can help you make sense of what's happening and can be an anchor. Also, one moment of revelation and insight won't change you. Instead, it's the change agent. It opens the possibility for greater change and healing to happen, but you still have to walk through the door, integrating and processing what was revealed to you.

We can't and won't tell you if plant-based healing will work for you, but it may be worth talking about with your therapist.

SACRED RITUALS AND CEREMONIES

As a child with grandparents who survived the Holocaust, Rabbi Arielle Hanien knew bad things can happen in this world. Her grandparents had met in a displaced persons' camp, and her mother was the first child her grandparents had before they made it out of Europe. Her mother grew up without grandparents, aunts, uncles, and cousins.

Rabbi Hanien eventually became a trauma therapist and clinical psychologist, but she understood historical and intergenerational trauma before she had the words to describe it. "I had the benefit, mostly through my mother's influence, of growing up in a tradition that has a very rich kind of awareness of trauma. Within the Jewish faith, ritual and story forms a fabric that teaches people how to have resiliency in the face of trauma, even in the face of what human beings can do to one another."[12]

Rabbi Hanien's grandfather died when she was a girl, but there is a story that her mother told during Passover seder about him that has stayed with Rabbi Hanien and informs much of her work today. As Rabbi Hanien recalled for us, "He used to take it upon himself to grate the bitter herbs for the Passover seder. What struck me then and moves me even now is that he would grate those bitter herbs until his eyes burned and the tears rolled down his cheeks, and he would eat them that way too.

"At that point in the Passover seder, his face would turn red; the pain was registering. It's not a religious obligation to experience pain when you eat these. They do tend to evoke that kind of physiological response, the burning. In our family, as in many families, usually that led us to say, 'get your water ready,' or 'get this sweet mixture of all the spring fruits that we're going to eat in a minute ready,' so that we'll be able to drown out the bitterness. My grandfather made sure that it registered."

Rabbi Hanien's grandfather suffered losses that were so unspeakable that his family only learned about them after he had died and they went through his paperwork. But Passover seder, which commemorates the Jews being freed from slavery and leaving Egypt, allowed Rabbi Hanien's grandfather to locate his pain and place his personal despair within a bigger redemption story to find "this fabric of meaning and collective narrative, so that there was a container for the immensity, even the infinity, of his grief."[13]

This one annual ritual allowed his tears to flow and evoked emotion that was already inside of him. It gave him the opportunity to integrate his ordeal. He could release the enormous pain in a way that wasn't overwhelming; in fact, it could have been quite healing.

There might be some traumas that we never make sense of or understand the cause. Maybe that's okay. Maybe we don't need to talk about them. Still, the pain remains buried until we find some outlet.

But maybe the outlet can come from a ritual or ceremony. It doesn't have to be religiously oriented, although it could. It just needs to be something that has meaning for you and that allows you the space to release some pain.

THE ROAD TO RECOVERY

Andrew knew he had to keep living, but he was in limbo. The catalyst for his transformation came one night while he sat by his 13-month-old son, who was recovering in the ICU after a major surgery. Andrew realized he had two options. He could continue following the military medical system's treatment or he could find an alternative path.

His military training kicked in. He needed to embrace his current level of pain, and then channel it, act on it, and use it in a way to improve his situation. In that moment, Andrew made a promise to himself and his son that three things would happen.

First, he would return to the man of his preinjury days. Second, he would find a way to come off all the medications. And finally, once Andrew had achieved these two missions, he would have a new one to fulfill. He was going to figure out how to turn around and help someone else heal and recover just like him.

This meant Andrew had to look for new answers, and since the traditional therapies and healing modalities weren't working, he had to be open to alternative therapies and healing modalities. Enter Dr. Mark L. Gordon and his work treating traumatic brain injuries (TBIs).

In a serendipitous encounter, Andrew got an email from Dr. Gordon after he had read an article about Andrew's situation. Dr. Gordon shared his philosophy for treating TBIs by reducing inflammation in the brain and body, and he explained how he was working with a number of combat vets who had remarkable results.

Andrew was blown away by Dr. Gordon's work, so he reached out to set up an appointment. First, Dr. Gordon ran a panel of comprehensive hormone tests that he had developed. Andrew, like most of Dr. Gordon's patients, was deficient in key hormones. After taking Andrew's lab results, a detailed physical exam, and his history, Dr. Gordon created a personalized protocol to replenish Andrew's hormones and reduce inflammatory chemicals in his body.

When he had started working with Dr. Gordon, Andrew had been taking more than 13 medications. His doctors had told him he'd be on them for the rest of his life. Shortly after Andrew began Dr. Gordon's protocol, his memory and moods improved. His speech and balance returned. He stopped drinking heavily and could sleep soundly. He also was able to come off his prescription medications.

Everything from his cognitive to behavioral to physiological issues slowly disappeared, and within months, he was back to feeling and acting like his old self. It was nothing short of a miracle.

Andrew's road to recovery didn't stop with Dr. Gordon either. Through the process of healing his brain injuries, he came to realize there was something inside being blocked that needed resolution. But he wasn't sure what. A Navy SEAL whom he respected suggested that he try MDMA-assisted psychotherapy, which acts as a stimulant and a hallucinogen. Andrew had never thought about using psychedelics, but he wanted to resolve whatever was inside, so he worked with someone trained in administering it.

It was the most profound and remarkable experience of his life.

MDMA allowed him to go back and relive some difficult situations that he had no conscious idea were stuck inside. He went back and resolved combat memories as if he was there in real time, but with a more detached, yet connected, perspective. Andrew saw the situation from his own perspective, but also everyone else's who was there. He could feel what they felt.

Through MDMA, Andrew was able to see that he had done everything he could and that sometimes situations shake out the way they do. It was a gift of resolution that he didn't even know he needed.

Five years after Andrew began his road to recovery with Dr. Gordon and MDMA, he remains symptom- and medication-free. In his words, he's "exponentially a better husband, father, and person," and he's performing just as good, if not better, than his preinjury days.

Andrew is also fulfilling the third promise he made to himself and his son—he's helping others to heal on their road to recovery. Andrew, and his brother, Adam, a former army Apache aviator, started the Warrior Angels Foundation. In partnership with Dr. Gordon, they've helped over 500 U.S. service members and veterans benefit from Dr. Gordon's unique treatment protocol.

Like Andrew, every patient has received a customized plan to help them heal. Through the Warrior Angels Foundation, Andrew has also worked tirelessly to bring greater awareness and attention to TBIs and their symptoms.

"What I thought was the worst thing in my life, turned out to be one of the best," Andrew told us.[14] "I think [my brain injuries and trauma are] absolutely a gift. Not only do I have this amazing family, I have an amazing mission. We've been able to help thousands of people understand their traumas, how to deal with them, and how to get better."

Andrew's extraordinary story reminds us that sometimes on the road to recovery, it can take a few stops before we find the right treatments, therapists, and doctors. We owe it to ourselves, though, to keep going, seeking, and searching for the right answers.

REFLECTIONS

Did any ancient practice pop for you? Did you feel drawn to: fine-tune your diet? Revisit the kinds of movement you do throughout the day? Spend more time in Mother Nature? Explore meditation or plant medicine? Learn more about sacred rituals and ceremonies? Ancient wisdom exists to help us heal and release long-held traumas. The tools and techniques we listed in this chapter are also powerful methods for building greater resiliency, which will help protect you from an unpredictable, uncontrollable world. Try to select one ancient therapy to explore and then add into your daily routine, then make note of how you feel before, during, and after using it.

SAGE WISDOM

"You are either cleaning your karma, or you're creating more with every thought, feeling, and experience your body's having. You're part of the solution, or you're part of the problem. The only way to be part of the solution is to have the skills, awareness, knowledge, and awakening to know how to care for yourself, care for your family, and care for your community, then you can make this world a better place."

—Dr. Carl Totton

CHAPTER 9

SELF-NURTURING PRACTICES

Danielle needed to find a new path to healing.

In her late 30s, she met and fell in love with the man of her dreams. They were married in less than a year. Ten years into their marriage, her husband was diagnosed with lung cancer. They did every conventional and alternative treatment they could, but after two years fighting the disease, he passed away.

Life with her husband had been fun and bright. They had traveled the world together. They both loved going out to eat, and cooking delicious, healthy meals at home. They were into yoga and considered themselves spiritually minded in the New Age tradition. They talked for hours about everything—their feelings, current events, movies—and never ran out of topics.

For Danielle, losing her husband meant losing the light in her world. When he died, it felt like she had too. For the next five years, Danielle lived on autopilot, going through the motions of life but feeling disconnected from everything and everyone.

She had tried working with different therapists, including grief counselors, but they didn't really help. Danielle went to a psychotherapist, but she didn't want to talk about or analyze her experiences, thoughts, or emotions. One therapist suggested guided meditation. Danielle hated it.

Danielle lost all desire to travel, go to yoga, or cook healthy meals. She lived on fast food, takeout, and a couple of glasses of wine every night. She hated how she was living.

Her sister would casually suggest that Danielle start dating again, that maybe getting out and meeting a new man could help. "Absolutely not," Danielle would say. She couldn't imagine connecting intimately with another man ever again. First, none would ever compare to her husband, and second, why would she risk the pain of losing someone she loved again?

But Danielle argued with herself. She knew that her husband would want her to experience life again, and a part of her did, but she also didn't know how. She didn't feel like herself. Up and down had gotten flipped, and she kind of hated herself for not being strong enough to get through it. Danielle was ashamed that she felt broken and dead inside.

All Danielle wanted was to hide, though she knew that wasn't the answer. But then, what was?

OUR TRIALS

Trauma can make us feel fractured, where we've lost all or parts of ourselves somewhere along the way.

But nothing has been lost. Maybe some parts of yourself are hiding, but they're just waiting for you to seek them out and bring them back. And if you do this, you will slowly build a bridge back to yourself with oneness, wholeness, and unity.

This is the most epic quest we may take in all of life, and it's the one that we'd argue is the most worthwhile. Because when you find your hidden pieces, and when you build a bridge back to yourself, your world will shift for the better, the healthier, and the brighter. You will feel alive. You will be connected to your inner life force— ignited, moved, and energized by it in ways you may have never experienced before.

Of course, you want this for your life. Who doesn't? It's not a question of if you want this, it's how do you get it? What will it take? What do you have to do to find yourself?

We've already looked at two key pieces of this puzzle: modern therapies, and ancient traditions and natural remedies. Now it's time for the third: *self-nurturing practices*. These practices consist of self-soothing to recognize and take care of our mental, emotional, physical, and spiritual needs.

For most of us battling trauma, self-nurturing is a foreign language. We don't know where to begin. No one taught us. We weren't taught how to self-nurture in school (although maybe we should have). And most of us grew up with parents who had no clue how to self-nurture themselves, let alone how to nurture their kids.

We have had few if any role models to show us how to feel safe in our bodies, self-regulate intense emotions like fear, move through negative feelings and thoughts, differentiate between safe or unsafe environments and people, or build healthy relationships.

And any conversation around self-nurturing and self-care has to address the elephant in the room. Many of us with hidden trauma hold devastating beliefs that we don't deserve anything good or pleasurable or safe in this world. We believe we don't deserve to feel loved, happy, respected, or at peace.

But you deserve all of this and more. You deserve to feel cared for, safe, appreciated, and honored. You deserve to be surrounded by people and in environments that support you, that love you, and that respect you. You deserve to wake up every morning connected to your life force and energized to meet the day.

This is your birthright.

You were born to experience all that is good, positive, and life-supporting in this world, and you were made to share it too. It's almost impossible to escape from this life without experiencing some kind of traumatic event. But it isn't a life sentence to pain, misery, sorrow, or heartache. We're meant to move through all the moments of our lives so we can return to our core—to our life force.

Self-nurturing tools help us meet and move through this challenge. In this chapter, we want to flip your (mis)perceptions on self-nurturing and self-care, and we're going to show you some of the most common and beneficial daily activities and lifestyle changes that you can make right now. We're talking about adopting creativity and the arts, finding a trusted community, discovering a spiritual connection, and shifting how we talk to ourselves.

But there is so much more that you can do. In fact, many of the practices we have already introduced are also powerful self-nurturing activities—eating healthy, spending time in nature, moving your body, meditating. The same goes with finding a therapy and therapist to work with. Every act that you take to help yourself recover and build your resiliency is an act of self-nurturing.

Self-nurturing isn't something anyone can give to us; it's a gift we give to ourselves.

We hope you are inspired to go on this adventure to learn about yourself, to find whatever hidden pieces may be out there, and to ultimately build the bridge back to yourself.

This is the journey for *you*.

When you learn what lights you up, calms your racing mind and heart, and heals and supports you, then you can consciously arrange your life, lifestyle, and the people in it around what makes you feel alive.

Practicing self-nurturing doesn't mean you have to overhaul your life ASAP. It's making one small adjustment to your daily routine—that's all you need to do. Over time, you can add more.

Pick the self-nurturing practice that interests you the most—start there and see how you feel after a week or two. In the end, it doesn't matter what you do; just take one small step toward yourself right now. That's all you have to do.

When you begin caring for yourself, you help to break the trauma chain gripping your family, community, and world. Trauma is contagious, spreading throughout generations and hitting everyone you come into contact with. But self-nurturing is also contagious. When you take care of yourself, you become very conscious about what's healthy and supportive versus what isn't. And it affects everyone within your circle.

You become mindful and deliberate about what you choose to do with your life, the environments you put yourself in, and the people you allow into your circles. All the life-supporting, self-affirming decisions you're making will get passed down to your children and grandchildren. You become the teacher for them that you never had.

How powerful is that?

You can break the chain of pain. Not just for your family, but for your friends, employees, boss, and everyone you come into contact with every day. Just think for a second what could happen if more people like you took this journey? What would the world look like? What would our experiences be? What would we build and create if we resolved our pain and regularly practiced self-nurturing?

The possibilities for your life and the world we're co-creating right now are endless. But they'll never be born into reality unless each of us is willing to find the hidden parts of ourselves, to make ourselves whole once more, through the art of self-nurturing.

As you explore self-nurturing, may you feel empowered and excited for this stage of your journey. May you feel inspired to build the bridge back to yourself, and may you feel curious about who you'll meet on the other side.

This is achievable. This is possible. You can do it. We believe in you.

EMBRACE CREATIVITY AND THE ARTS

In Chapter 7, we talked about how you can use expressive art therapies to help resolve your trauma. The good news is that you can use them all the time by adding them into your daily (or at least regular) self-nurturing routine.

You have a lot of choices on the medium you can use. Painting, drawing, sculpting, making collages, writing, dancing, playing, and listening to music are only a few. You don't need formal training either. You could go to the store right now, buy markers, a blank pad of paper, and start drawing.

Art helps us find a way to make our pain visible and to express everything we're feeling and thinking in a safe and healthy way, rather than stuffing, storing, and ignoring it.

Through art, we also reconnect to our inner child—the one who may be really wounded, who's scared and may be hiding from all the trauma we endured growing up. As we engage in art, we build the bridge to our inner child. We create the safe space for that part of ourselves to come out from hiding and to have fun again.

This alone is healing and can help us loosen our tight, fear-driven nervous system response to the world. When we have fun, we relax. Our anxiety goes down. Our minds can stop racing.

We can also get into flow, which is when time and space seem to converge and inner energy and strength move us. We're communicating from the inside out and creating from our heart and soul.

We may have revelations and insights that leave us going, "That was so good! Where did that come from?"

With art, *you* get to choose everything, from the medium you use to what you create. Trauma can leave us feeling disempowered and out of control. Art helps us to feel empowered in a safe environment.

There's one more amazing turn that happens with art, and it's the slow move from dark, deep pain into the light. In one story we were told, a woman had started to draw in a blank journal. She had never drawn before and certainly didn't consider herself an artist. She grabbed a black magic marker and started scribbling. She went all the way back into her past, beginning with her childhood when she had been neglected by her parents. She didn't have the words to describe what she was feeling—which is common when trauma happens to us as kids.

Instead, she just scribbled away. At first her marks were dark and heavy, where she pressed her marker down hard in the journal. Then she drew a picture of herself standing and looking over her shoulder with chains around her neck, arms, and feet.

Week by week, she kept drawing, filling her journal with scribbles and sketches of her past, and over time they became lighter. She eventually switched from using a black marker to green and blue ones.

She felt lighter after every entry, where the scribbles helped her to release her stored pain.

So, what would art as self-nurturing look like in your daily routine?

It might be writing or drawing in a journal. Maybe you write letters to your trauma, your younger self, the event that happened, or the person who harmed you. You're not sending these, you're simply using them as a container to pour your thoughts and feelings into without censoring yourself, because whatever you're feeling is what matters most and *nothing* you feel is wrong.

It could be that you paint with acrylics, pastels, or watercolors. It could be sculpting or working with clay. It could be writing a novel, play, or short essay if that moves you. Not that you need to share or publish these works; you only need a container to put your lived experiences into.

It could also be improvised dancing. Put on some gentle or upbeat music—whatever moves you (no pun intended)—and let your body lead you. No one's watching, so you can do whatever silly moves you're guided to. Wave your arms. Kick your legs. Twist or bend any which way, shake those hips, and laugh while you do it. (Just be careful. If you haven't moved your body in a while like this, don't go to town, yanking or straining a muscle.)

Maybe you want to enter through music. Maybe you play an instrument, or you write a song. You could even listen to instrumental music or nature sounds like rain falling or ocean waves, or whatever strikes you in the heart chord and pours from you into an external expression of your soul.

We could keep listing ways to practice self-nurturing through art, but we'll let you take it from here. Be creative. Find what feels right for you. Art is about creating and unleashing your power within. However it happens and whatever the end product looks like is up to you. There's no right or wrong here.

The more you do this, the more you will find that not only is it a way to free yourself from your past, it becomes a way for you to make sense of your experiences today. We will still face challenging moments, and we'll need tools and practices that help us move past these events. Art can be a wonderful tool to help you, no practice necessary.

Find Your Unique Activities

A huge part of self-nurturing is about discovering what's fun and pleasurable to you. What do you love to do? What makes you feel alive, engaged, joyful, or any positive, life-giving emotion? Be creative. Find your unique happy zone. Let your heart and emotions guide you. Try different activities too. Learn about yourself and have fun with this.

To get you out of the gate, here are some activities that the experts we spoke to use in their self-nurturing practices.

- Limiting negative media
- Taking social media breaks
- Eating healthy
- Exercising daily
- Gardening
- Spending time in nature
- Reading uplifting books
- Cooking and/or baking
- Taking a bath with scented water or bubbles
- Making lavender water and homemade herbal teas
- Traveling solo (including other parts of your city/town, neighboring states, domestically, or internationally)
- Taking online classes
- Going to yoga or the gym
- Meeting a close friend for tea/coffee, in person
- Gazing at the stars and moon in the night sky
- Crocheting, knitting, or sewing
- Hiking, biking, or kayaking/canoeing
- Watching movies that bring joy
- Making pottery
- Making jewelry
- Wood working
- Photography
- Organizing home clutter

FIND YOUR COMMUNITY

When we are in pain or have been wounded, it's natural to want to retreat inward. We want to go into our shells and protect our wounded hearts and selves. Sometimes we need to take a time-out from the world and people. But doing so can turn into isolation.

Humans need connection and social interactions. We also need to feel safe, but trauma often leaves us feeling anything but. Hence, we distance. We lock ourselves away. It takes time and practice to learn, possibly for the first time, how to feel safe, especially with other people.

We're going to say the quiet part out loud. *You won't feel safe with everyone.* There are just some people in our lives who are negative. They pull us down with their attitudes, judgments, and behaviors. They may be unsupportive, or they may make mean, belittling, snide comments to us.

The truth is some people don't belong in our lives. As you take this road to recovery, you may find "friends" who fall away. You may find that your relationships with people shift without you meaning for them too. And you may find that you consciously start choosing who to spend your time with, acknowledging that some people are just unhealthy.

Often, we need to find new communities and people to connect with. Maybe it's a shared interest like a yoga class or a book club, or it could be a group connected to trauma, such as a community art, dance, or music therapy program or support group. You're looking for a place where you can immerse yourself in safe, healthy, and healing connections with others.

Part of these connections come from being able to speak about your trauma—eventually—to *safe witnesses*. These are the people who aren't intimidated by your pain or what you've been through. They can listen without judgment and bear witness to your experiences. Sometimes that person is a therapist; other times it's a trusted friend and ally you meet.

Having our traumas witnessed is one of the great keys to healing and releasing your inner anger, shame, and difficult emotions. "One of the critical factors of anger, self-blame, and shame is that you're so embarrassed or humiliated by the trauma, so much that you don't talk about it," explained Jodi Cohen, a nutritional therapy practitioner.[1]

Cohen, who lost her 12-year-old son in a tragic car accident, credits her friends as being incredible support for her in the weeks, months, and years after the accident as she processed her grief and learned how to be a single mother while helping her 14-year-old daughter through the trauma too. "When we can speak what's on our mind to someone who we feel safe with, it helps us to process the experience too," Cohen told us.[2] "In speaking those words, it releases the trauma from your body and allows you to flourish and not be stuck."[3]

Finding the people who we can let down our guards with and talk through whatever sticky challenges we're having is one of the most self-nurturing gifts we can give ourselves for our recovery and beyond.

Yes, it does take some vulnerability. It may mean you have to be the one to go first and strike up a conversation, invite someone for coffee or a walk, or simply to share what you've been going through. But you may be pleasantly surprised what a little initiative turns into. Stephanie Speights, an eco-spiritual practitioner in Los Angeles, decided one day that she wanted to know her neighbors. She had lived in the same apartment for 25 years and had watched kids in diapers go off to college, but she didn't know their names. She started to realize that she knew people's cars more than the drivers themselves.

This wasn't how she wanted to live, so one day she knocked on about 30 doors and invited everyone to her house. "I was nervous, so I used the word *we*, because that made me feel more empowered, like 'we want to invite you to this event.' About ninety-five percent of the people went 'Oh my God, thank you so much for doing this. I've wanted to, but I've been too afraid that people would say no and not show up.'"[4]

This one gathering turned into an ongoing, regular coming together called "alley up." They've done potlucks, neighborhood tomato plantings, art exhibits, and more. People hug each other on the street. They pet sit each other's cats and dogs. They have a community spirit and connection that happened because one person said, "Let's do it."

"It was really an exercise in moving through the fear with the goal of human connection," Stephanie told us. "I wanted my outside life to be more fulfilled."[5]

People want connections—not the shallow ones that breed negativity. We yearn for honest, authentic, and real human connections.

There are more people out there craving this, needing this in their lives, just like you. You are not alone. And when you find these people, and this community, it can open up your life in miraculous ways.

BUILD A SPIRITUAL COMMUNITY

Our minds are powerful problem-solvers. They seek patterns, weaving together elaborate stories about the way the world works and why some experiences happen to us, devising clever ways to keep us "safe."

When it comes to grappling with emotions, our minds often get us in trouble. We have to stop thinking and learn to listen to our inner voice, the wise and timeless one. To quiet our mind, sometimes we have to bring in something that is beyond it, bigger than any one person.

We're talking about the Divine, God, Allah, the Universe, the Great Mystery, the Life Force, or any name that feels right to you. It's the higher power that animates the world and moves all living things. Since time began, civilizations have had different names for the thousands of faces they've created to explain the Divine.

Trauma often disconnects us from the source of all that is. But if we can find our way back, it will help us to create a foundation on which we can order our lives and move through the world, facing anything and everything that we encounter.

Faith in something bigger and higher than ourselves can give us strength to look at our resentments, anger, and suffering. It can help us make sense of the world, our place in it, and how we choose to move forward from this day until our last. It restores hope and inspiration and reminds us that this world has both the dark and the light, the bad and the good, the selfish and the selfless.

"Spiritual healing is often looked at as the most profound healing that we can give ourselves," explained Darcy Lubbers, a board-certified clinical art therapist and marriage and family therapist. "As we connect to all aspects of who we are—physical, emotional, mental, spiritual beings—we can shift our perspective and foster a sense of who we are at our essence and what our connection is to other beings in this universe."[6]

What does it mean to have a spiritual practice that self-nurtures? How do we figure out what it means, especially when we may still be reeling from our traumas? How do we move through anger, bitterness, and rage at the Divine because of what we've suffered?

For some of us, it can be hard to move through that and reach a place where we can believe in a force that's loving, kind, and compassionate. Let's face it, there is so much pain and suffering and, yes, darkness with some terrible acts in this world that it can feel too hard to walk the path back to the Divine.

Several of the experts we spoke to said that many people go through periods of being agnostic. If you're at that place, it's okay.

You may find that as you release some of the trauma through other therapies that feeling lighter, and maybe happier, slowly brings you closer to the Divine or your life force. It's hard to stay disconnected when you are able to experience true joy, gratitude for life, and peace within yourself.

Meditation can also help lead you to your source. When we silence our mind chatter, we go within and we learn to listen, observe, and witness ourselves while connecting to our core. As we connect to our core, it's really hard to remain distant from a higher power. Your heart and soul will reemerge, reopening to the wonder and awe of this life, planet, and your existence.

Spending time in nature is another key to unlocking your life force within. Sensing the beauty that is Mother Earth, seeing her leaves, rocks, and trees, feeling the wind, watching birds and other animals go about their days—all of this can generate that sense of awe and wonder. Slowly, your heart will crack open to the other side of suffering.

Self-nurturing activities like creating art, music, or writing can also unlock that door. You may discover that it's not you who finds the Divine, but the Divine who finds you. And you may find that the Universe and life force within you never really left you—it was just waiting for you to remember and become ready for the connection once more.

You've probably noticed that we've differentiated between organized religion and spirituality. That's on purpose. Connecting to a spiritual practice doesn't have to come through a church, synagogue, or mosque. If it does, that's perfectly all right. If your path leads you elsewhere, that's perfectly all right too.

Let your heart call the shots. It will steer you in the right direction.

SHIFT HOW YOU TALK TO YOURSELF

Trauma can create harmful beliefs that rule our lives. Most of the time, we don't even know they exist. "I'm unlovable," or "No one will ever love me," or "I'm unworthy," or "I'll never amount to anything," or "I deserved it," or "It's all my fault" are some examples of the infectious beliefs we absorb about ourselves and the world.

The earlier these were formed, the harder they can be to find. When we experienced "Little t" traumas, it can be especially tough finding the hook. We legitimately may have no memory. There may not be anything we can trace our trauma all the way back to. Yet we know something is off because we see it in our lives. It might show up as self-sabotage of our own success, finances, or health.

How do we solve for this?

According to Patrick Gentempo, DC, it's through affirmations, but not the ones where we repeat to ourselves, "I am wealthy. I am abundant." When trauma is in the picture, positive affirmations often flop. That's because deep down, we don't believe them.

Let's say you're broke and in debt, and you've struggled with it all your adult life. If you say, "I am wealthy. I am abundant," it will create a dissonance inside. You'll say the words, but you'll feel broke and poor, and you'll feel like you're lying to yourself about your reality.

Instead, we need to add two key words to our affirmations: "I choose . . ."

I choose wealth.　　　　　*I choose peace.*
I choose abundance.　　　*I choose safety.*
I choose to be fit and healthy.　*I choose respect.*
I choose to be loved.

"What I'm saying is, 'Maybe I didn't make that choice in the past, but I'm going to make that for my future. I choose something new for my future,'" explained Dr. Gentempo.[7]

Where affirmations have gone amuck is where people are walking around saying, "I'm happy. I'm happy," when they're not. "I choose happiness" means "okay, I might not be happy right this second, but I choose it, and I'm going to start moving toward it."

Switching our affirmations slightly, saying them first thing in the morning and in a clear, powerful, intentional voice, makes a strong statement to yourself. You're bridging the distance between your inner self and your experience in the outer world.

If you want to kick it up a notch, do what's called *mirror work*. It's a tool many of our experts have their patients use. You stand in the mirror, look yourself in the eyes, and say, "I love you."

Sometimes it's hard to see what stares back at us. We harbor so many negative self-images, self-talk, and low self-esteem what we can't look at ourselves in the mirror. And if that's something that's tough for you, first, know that you're not alone, and second, recognize it's a powerful knowledge. It shows that you're internally out of balance. You can correct this through continued mirror work and/or under the watchful guidance of a trusted therapist.

In the beginning, it can feel painful to speak in a caring, loving, kind way to ourselves. In many ways, it's alien. The culture we live in has repeatedly focused us on our flaws, telling us to fix our looks, bodies, and wealth.

Yes, we can adopt healthier, more self-nurturing practices so we can take even better care of our minds, bodies, hearts, and souls, but fundamentally there's nothing *wrong* with you. Your perception of yourself and how you feel about you needs some adjusting, that's all. When you do this, then some of the self-care activities you need to resolve your trauma will naturally fall into place because you want to do them.

You want to take better care of yourself. Often, it starts by making small adjustments, then some more, and then some more, and before you realize it, you're like the caterpillar who's turned into the butterfly—you've transformed your life in dramatic ways.

This will take some deep digging and a willingness to shed what no longer works. But over time, it will change your life.

THE ROAD TO RECOVERY

Art was Danielle's answer.

Danielle used to love journaling but had stopped after her husband died. For her birthday, a friend gifted her a journal. One night, Danielle curled up in her favorite chair and started writing in it. The entry was short, but there was something about holding the pen and the journal in her hands that made her feel peaceful and content. It was brief, but it felt right to her.

From then on, she began journaling every night before she went to sleep. At first, she only wrote about what she did daily, then that gave way to writing about her feelings in the moment and during the day. Slowly, her entries shifted to other feelings and thoughts surrounding her husband's death and what life now looked like for her. Some nights, tears came—a lot of them—but she kept writing through them.

Weeks, then months, went by, and while she wouldn't say she was healed or recovered, she was feeling better. She started reading poetry too, and found the words spoke to her on a deep soul level. Soon poems mixed into her journal entries. It grew into a ritual that she looked forward to at the end of each day.

Danielle would brew a cup of mint tea, turn on instrumental music, light a few candles, and pull out her poetry books and journal, letting whatever needed releasing come out onto the page. It freed something inside of her as she processed her grief and trauma, and worked to make sense of life and her place in it. She traveled back in time to her childhood, exploring how she never felt like she fit into her family. She wrote about her strained relationship with her mother, whom she felt had been judgmental and controlling, and her father, whom she never felt she had a connection with. As she understood her family dynamics, it clarified why her relationship with her husband had been so monumental in her life.

From writing, Danielle found her way to a movement therapy class. She had never taken a dance class before, but through her journaling she realized that she needed to find a new version of life for herself. She vowed to try different activities. Dancing calmed her, and it was another outlet for her to express her emotions.

Through dance, she reconnected to her body. She was surprised to find how much trauma and pain she had stored in it. As she moved, she could feel her emotions rise—the fear, sadness, loneliness, and sense of abandonment.

Danielle spent the next three years reconnecting to herself and processing her experience of losing her husband. Her road to recovery wasn't instantaneous—none really are—but she felt transformed. Through writing and dance, she found the parts of herself that had gotten locked away, and she started to put herself back together in a different way.

Today, Danielle travels again. She takes solo trips, and she's gone on a couple of organized ones. She still journals and writes poetry, and she dances regularly and found she loves the tango. She's back to cooking healthy meals and taking care of her body.

She's even told her sister that she thinks she may be ready to start dating. She's not in a rush, but the idea of connecting again doesn't terrify her as it once did. There are still days and certain times of the year when she misses her husband and her pain resurfaces, but she recognizes it. She'll journal about it, call her sister or a close friend, go for a bike ride, or work in the garden, another activity she discovered she really enjoys.

She now has tools she can use to help her explore and move through whatever intense emotion or experience comes into her life. In the end, that's all any of us can ask for, really. We don't and can't control what happens in our lives, but we can control how we respond to and what we do with them.

REFLECTIONS

Did you find something new to try, or did you remember an activity that you once did that felt nurturing? Now is the time to sit and consider what *one* practice you can bring into your life today. Could it be embracing creativity and the arts—music, writing, dancing? Could it be expanding to find a new, healthier, and more supportive community? Could it be exploring and finding a deeper spiritual connection? Could it be working on talking to yourself in a kinder way? Whatever you choose, it will be right for you. No need to justify. Ask yourself, *What do I need?*, then pay attention to the first response. Often, that's our body-mind-heart connection answering us. Whatever you answer, add it to your life and notice how it affects you. Keep track of how you feel before, during, and after you use one. Self-nurturing practices should nurture you, leaving you feeling better, stronger, and more relaxed. If they don't, then they may not be the right ones for you to use, or the right ones for you now. Either way, they provide powerful information that you need to help you make the best, most informed choices about your road to recovery.

SAGE WISDOM

"There's a part of us inside—our essence, our soul—that wasn't damaged by the abuse. It went underground. This part of us is beautiful, radiant, and you might not know it's there. Part of the healing process is to rediscover it and to realize 'you're not bad, not wrong, and not terrible,' but instead, you're this beautiful soul."

—Dr. Margaret Paul

CHAPTER 10

LOVE, BOUNDARIES, AND FORGIVENESS

Jenny didn't recognize the person in the mirror.

A former Division I cross-country ski racer, a marathon runner, and now a mother, Jenny was known as the "fun mom," always doing activities, having playdates, putting on dinner parties, volunteering, and saying yes to everything and everyone.

In her late 20s, she loved her life.

That's why she felt so blindsided when the strange physical symptoms appeared—the extreme fatigue, the swelling, the brain fog. Eventually, she learned that she had four strains of Lyme disease that were in her brain stem, spinal cord, and nervous system. She also had hundreds of parasites in her body that had put holes in her organs and endocrine glands. And when the parasites died, they released viruses, bacteria, and neurotoxins into her body.

In six months, Jenny gained 70 pounds—mostly from the massive amounts of toxins. Her liver and kidneys couldn't process the toxins fast enough, so her body used the survival mechanism of creating fat to store the toxins and keep them away from her organs.

Jenny's body was under siege, and no one knew how to fix it.

For two years, Jenny watched as her body grew weaker. She felt chronically stressed—mentally, physically, emotionally, and spiritually. Making it worse, Jenny and her husband discovered a massive mold outbreak in their home. The mold had caused chronic health issues for their daughter, who once had such a severe allergic reaction that she almost had to be life-flighted out. Their home had to be renovated, but it wasn't easy. The family moved six times, staying with Jenny's parents, camping, and living in small cabins.

What more could happen? Jenny wondered. The stress of everything was so intense that she felt like her nervous system had been hijacked. She tried meditating, something that had always helped, but it didn't now. She tried positive affirmations, but they felt hollow. Forget running—that was out of the question. But even slow walks in nature and gentle yoga were too much.

Although she barely had the energy or strength to get out of bed, Jenny still tried to muscle through, showing up for her kids and saying yes to her normal routine. But it was all too much. One day, she crawled under the covers in her bed and curled up into a ball.

Her husband tried to help her feel better. "You can do this," he told her encouragingly.

But she disagreed. "No, I've tried. I've been trying for years, and it's not working. I've gone *beyond the point where I can return.*"

The disease, the parasites, the entire two-year ordeal had stolen everything from her—her energy, outlook, health, identity, and now her life.

As she lay in bed, her thoughts spun to the future. *Will my life ever be the same? Why is this happening to me? Am I going to be bedridden for the rest of my life? Will I ever be able to play with my children or meet a friend for a walk again? Will I ever work? What kind of life is this?*

Jenny was overwhelmed. She couldn't live the day-to-day life she had loved. She wasn't sure if getting it back was even possible, and if it wasn't, then what was in store for her future?

OUR TRIALS

Have you ever wondered, *What's wrong with me? Why am I not over my trauma by now?*

Do you feel frustrated and confused, angry and disappointed, because you can't stick with a self-nurturing practice? Are the therapies you're using not working or not working fast enough?

Are you constantly giving more of yourself—your time, energy, mind, body, heart, soul—than everyone else in your life?

Do you ever ask, *When does this pain and torment end? When do I get to find peace?*

On this trauma journey, our final stop is the answer to all of these questions that haunt everyone. We're talking about *self-love.*

Trauma has a way of cutting us off from self-love and causing us to feel the opposite, self-hate. We may believe that we're dirty, wrong, bad, shameful, guilty, ugly, unworthy, less than, or unlovable—all the same scripts we've talked about that hold us back from embracing self-nurturing practices. Most of us have hugely critical voices in our heads, judging ourselves constantly. These insidious voices whisper that we're not "getting over our traumas fast enough," that we're "not being disciplined enough to exercise or meditate," that we'll "never change or get better," and that we're "so weak-willed it's pathetic."

For all of this harsh self-talk, nothing is further from the truth. You are incredible. You are a survivor. From the moment trauma first struck your life, you have done everything you possibly could to keep yourself alive. You are strong and smart. You are intuitive and proud. You are good and right, worthy and deserving. *You* are lovable.

Self-love means feeling appreciation, gratitude, and awe for *you*— for every traumatic experience that you've endured, for who you've become, and for the life that you're now consciously creating. You can't force yourself to feel this, but you can help it along. Every therapy, therapist, ancient wisdom, natural remedy, and self-nurturing practice that you embrace is actually an act of self-love.

Now, in this chapter, we're covering the final two essential ingredients: setting healthy boundaries and finding forgiveness.

We're not taught how to do either, but both are powerful practices that help us unwind our traumas, create more resiliency for the future, and ultimately arrive at self-love. In this chapter, we're getting clear on *what* setting healthy boundaries and finding forgiveness means, *why* they're so important, and *how* you can support them in your life. We're sharing some exercises that the trauma experts we spoke to use with their patients, so you get a sense for how therapists and healers can support you in this work. If you want to try these practices on your own, go for it. If it's too much or too intense as solo excursions, then please reach out to a professional.

We know that we keep hammering in that point, but it's so important. So many of us live life believing we have to do this on our own, when that's not the case. There are incredible allies who want to help you, and they can if we let them. Sometimes getting the courage to ask for help is the hardest part, but it's so worth taking that step.

Here's the secret: Self-love isn't something you have to create. It's already within you. It's just waiting for you to open that door, even if it's just a crack. It takes a willingness and courage to let yourself feel it, and if you do, your life will shift and change in positive, life-affirming, life-supporting ways.

You deserve this.

As you go through this leg of your quest, may you start to awaken to how amazing you are. May you begin to feel—even if it's for a moment—that you are deserving and worthy of living a life filled with joy, appreciation, strength, pleasure, excitement, energy, and love.

SETTING HEALTHY BOUNDARIES

People who love themselves set healthy boundaries.

They have the ability to know what is acceptable in their lives and can say, "No, I will not allow this." We all need boundaries. They help us to know who we are, how we feel, and what we're thinking, and they are what we need to stay centered, healthy, and filled with our life force.

Boundaries show us who we want to be, how we want to be treated, and the experiences we want to have in the world.

Unfortunately, many people with unresolved trauma have no idea what boundaries are, how to set them, or that they are allowed for themselves. That's partly due to our culture. No one teaches us about boundaries. For women, it's more complicated. It's often expected that they put aside their needs and sense of self for others, especially when children come into the picture.

The other part has to do with trauma. Those of us who have experienced childhood trauma often lack boundaries to begin with. We were never allowed to have them. We had no ability or agency in our lives to tell someone to stop. We couldn't speak up to say what was okay—we probably didn't even know what "okay" felt like.

Or we may have learned to doubt ourselves. If our trauma has been dismissed or downplayed, say we have constantly been told that we're "oversensitive," or "stop being a baby," or we had a parent who continually criticized or was mean to us, then we could have been disconnected from our perception of reality. Boundaries would have become confusing, where we have no idea what "safe" feels like.

If trauma slammed into your life as an adult, it will have changed you on so many levels. You will now have to relearn boundaries (assuming you had a firm hold on them before). There is a very real "before and after" feel to your life, so what may have been acceptable previously may not be anymore—or vice versa.

Regardless of your trauma, you need healthy boundaries.

Without them, you can lose your sense of self. You may care more about keeping harmony and peace in a relationship—whether that's in your personal or professional life—becoming a "people pleaser." And when you continually push aside your emotions and needs, you can be more vulnerable to being taken advantage of or exploited.

The fallout? You say yes at work when you really don't have the energy, time, or capacity to take on more. You fill your social calendar when you're exhausted and burned out. You spend time with people who bring you down instead of lifting and supporting you. In the end, you give so much of yourself, time, energy, and love to the people in your world, but you never receive the same.

This isn't a path to happiness. It's a straight shot to resentment, bitterness, anger, and despair. Instead of meaningful, deep, and supportive relationships, you create a world where people keep hurting you because you don't believe you deserve anything better.

It can also set you up for more trauma. "People who can say no and establish a boundary can hold on to their sovereignty and who they are," explained Dr. Yvonne Farrell, an acupuncturist and doctor of Oriental medicine.[1] "If you are comfortable in who you are, then many traumatic experiences are not going to impact you in the same way, and you'll be able to manage them better."[2]

Learning to create boundaries also helps to resolve trauma. You will feel safer when you set and acknowledge what's healthy for you. You'll also learn to trust yourself, as you prove that you can take care of you.

Setting healthy boundaries will exponentially improve your relationships. People who love and care about you will want to respect your boundaries. It may take some uncomfortable conversations with the people you love about why you need these boundaries and how you want to be supported, especially if you've never set them in the past. But the people who truly matter will stand by you.

You'll also find out if there are some people who no longer fit into your life. Maybe someone who you have loved can't meet your needs. Whatever the reasons may be, you'll be faced with a decision as to whether this relationship is important enough to find a way forward or if it's time to let it go. This may be a hard realization to come to.

But generally, when you set boundaries, you get to show up as the best version of yourself, whether that's as a parent, spouse, partner, employee, boss, co-worker, friend, sibling, child, grandparent, you name it.

All of this being said, we know how hard it can be to set a boundary, moreover to identify what you need. We also want to acknowledge that for people who have survived sexual and physical abuse, setting boundaries can feel especially terrifying. We want you to know that whatever emotions pop up around boundaries, they're valid and real, and it's okay.

Setting boundaries is hard, especially if you've never lived that way. Still, you deserve to have them and they're healthy. To help you get started, we've included some of the most common practices that the trauma experts we spoke to use with their patients. If it feels right for you, try them. If you meet a lot of resistance or it feels hard, there is no shame in reaching out for a little assistance.

Most of the therapists and experts we spoke with teach and work on this skill with all their patients. Like everything in life, please be kind and gentle with yourself.

Practice Self-Awareness

To have healthy boundaries, we have to know ourselves. This takes self-awareness. We have to tap into how we feel and what we need physically, emotionally, mentally, and spiritually. There's no wrong answer, but it means going inward and constantly checking in with yourself to assess how you're doing and the environment and people around you. You'll want to ask yourself, "What am I sensing and feeling? How are people treating me? Are they treating me in a positive, kind, and well-intentioned way, or are they trying to be hurtful to me?"

Adding self-nurturing practices into your life can go a long way to help you connect with yourself. These practices can teach you what is good, pleasurable, and healing for your mind, body, heart, and soul. This isn't an overnight success story but a journey that will span your lifetime. That's a good thing. We're constantly evolving and transforming.

The more you go inward and become curious about observing your experience, the easier it becomes to find your limits. For instance, if you're snapping at your kids and have a short fuse with your spouse, then that's usually a sign something is off. You're the only one who can figure out the why. It could be that you're pulled in too many directions and you need to find at least 30 minutes a day just for you. Maybe the answer comes through meditating or journaling or from having an open conversation with your spouse about how you're feeling, or maybe you call a close friend or a therapist who could talk it out with you and help you process.

How you get to the answer and what "it" is could be anything. The key is that you're aware something is off, that it needs addressing, and that you're the one who takes responsibility to find what you need, set the boundary, and stand behind it.

As you discover who you are, you begin valuing yourself, which makes it impossible to stay quiet. You *have to* voice what you need. You *have to* put a boundary in place. You *have to* stand by you. The more you do this, the easier it becomes. Think of it as a muscle that needs strengthening. The more you practice, the stronger it becomes.

Know Your Values

Sometimes it's hard to know what's important. When we go inward, what are we looking for? Hunt for your values, which will tell you so much about who you are, who you want to be, and what and who you want in your life.

Values are the deeply held beliefs that are the core of who we are, how we see the world, and how we want to experience it. Respect, honesty, trust, fairness, listening, cooperation, kindness, compassion, openness, love—we all have values. We're just not always conscious of them.

When we aren't, it's easy for our boundaries to get eroded. For instance, if it's important that you're heard and listened to, but people in your life consistently cut you off when you're talking, dismiss what you have to say, or aren't listening, then every time that happens, it's a dagger in your chest.

This isn't how you want to live. When you know you value being heard and listened to, then you're able to create that boundary that says, "Hey, it feels very hurtful and disrespectful when I'm interrupted. When I'm talking, can you please let me finish?" If they continue to interrupt, then you get to act. You can say, "If I'm interrupted, the conversation will end" or whatever choice feels better for you.

This sounds scary, right? When you're not used to standing up for yourself, it can feel like you're jumping off a cliff. But the more you practice and know your values, the more it will become second nature.

We know how frustrating experiences and people can be. You may feel like you don't have many—if any—choices. If it's your boss, you may feel like you can't have this conversation or that there's nothing you can do to change how they treat you. While that may be true, you still can shift how *you* see the world.

Your perception and attitude have power.

Maybe you realize that working for someone who values what you have to say is really important. If you can't change your boss, maybe you look for another job working for someone who better aligns with how you want to be treated. Or maybe you realize that it's hard to talk face to face—your boss may struggle to listen—so instead you decide to write an email so your ideas can be heard. Or maybe you realize that when you spoke up in the past, your voice was timid and soft, so you shift slightly to speak more assertively and powerfully, holding eye contact with your back straight and chin up.

There will always be people and events outside our control—that's life. But we control our reactions—our emotions, thoughts, and behaviors. Every time you tap into your values and stand by them, you step into your inner strength. Every time someone violates what you value, you will know it. And instead of throwing up your hands and saying, "Well, that's life. I can't control them, so I'll just sit here and take it," you will proactively stand up for yourself.

Every time you do this, you learn that you can trust yourself. That you have agency over your life. That you are powerful and strong and no matter what happens in the external world, no matter what someone says or does, *you* will take care of it.

This is how you build resiliency in life. You take back control over your body, mind, heart, and soul. No one can touch them. And you teach yourself that you will, and can, take care of you.

That being said, we do have to acknowledge that there are some situations and people where standing up for yourself can put you in danger. We're talking about domestic violence or experiences at work that could threaten your job security. While we absolutely want you to hold true to your values, do it safely and in a time frame that is right for you.

This may require you to seek outside help from a domestic violence support network or a trusted therapist who can help you create a plan for yourself (and your children, if they're involved). Sometimes it may mean walking away from a harmful work environment, never saying anything to your boss (or a co-worker if that's the source).

Just know that you have the right to set healthy boundaries, and you are the only one who gets to decide what these look like.

Wall Work

As Dr. Sam Rader, a psychologist, told us, sometimes when we've experienced trauma, especially if we had to go limp and play possum, we experience a sense of ourselves as a beta pack animal. We're not the strong alpha leaders. Instead, we're submissive and we don't feel we can protect ourselves or be strong.

In nature, beta animals have inhibitory mechanisms in the brains that prevent any aggressive impulse from being completed. If we're living like betas, our brains won't let us say no or fight back.

But you can override this control center.

"If you think that you are a submissive pack animal, and you have these inhibitory mechanisms, it's very hard to push past that fear, that shame, that guilt and come into your power and uprightness," Dr. Rader explained.[3] "But if you can push past the inhibition, you are telling your brain that it is safe to express aggression. In nature, if there's a submissive pack animal who one day has the courage to override the inhibitory mechanisms and actually confront an alpha animal, if they have that fight, it does not matter whether they win or lose, from that day forward the beta is regarded as an alpha in the pack."[4]

"They change their brains, and they change their status in the community. We're the same as those animals. If we are able to stand, feel our muscles, feel our power, feel our ability to say no, then we are able to carry ourselves like an alpha and change how it feels to be inside of our bodies and how people react to us in the world."[5]

To help patients push past their inhibitions, Dr. Rader uses a practice from somatic experiencing called *Wall Work*, where they push against a wall as hard as they can, screaming, growling, and grunting like an animal. This retrains their brain that it's okay to defend and show aggression.

Now, no one is saying that you should start a fight or get physical. It's just teaching your mind that you do have the power to stand up for and protect yourself and that you hold the authority in your life.

Build Your "No" Muscle

Just practicing saying no can help you override your beta programming. Think about how often you say this two-letter word. Does the thought alone make you feel guilty or bad? It's okay if it does; that's common.

Start easy. Just say no to yourself in the mirror. Say it to the easiest person in your life—someone who you know is 100 percent in your corner and supportive, nonjudgmental, and totally understanding, always.

Or the next time someone asks you to do something, say, "Let me think about it. I'll get back to you." This is one of the greatest responses you can give. It's a check on all the reflexive yeses that you may give when you really don't have the time, energy, or capacity. When you say, "I'll get back to you," it's a boundary. It allows you to check in with yourself when you're in a quieter, more relaxed space. When you have the answer, then you can email, text, or call.

Think of this as building your "no" muscle. Take actions that are slightly out of your comfort zone, and over time, setting boundaries will become easier.

If getting to "no" remains difficult, it could be a sign you need to look within. Often it's unconscious beliefs and fears—usually created because of our traumas—that stop us from acting in our own best interests.

You may need to ask some uncomfortable questions like "What do I think is going to happen if I say no? Why would I rather please people than myself? Does it go back to childhood? Am I a caretaker of everyone else but me? Why do I believe someone else's feelings and experience are more important than mine?"

We'll admit, these are deep, profound questions, but if you can look in the mirror and be honest with yourself, the answers can transform you. If you need an outside assist from a therapist or healer, please welcome it. They can help you see clearly what often gets distorted or hidden.

FINDING FORGIVENESS

Now we come to our final act. Finding forgiveness.

The word *forgiveness* gets batted around a lot in trauma circles. It's essential when it comes to resolving our pain, but it's also one of the most widely misunderstood spiritual and psychological practices. Most of us are programmed to think forgiveness is a way of telling the person (we'll call them the perpetrator) that what they did is okay, or that we "forgive them" for what they did. If there isn't another person involved—say it's a natural disaster, accident, or a pandemic—then it's forgiving God, the Divine, the Universe, Life that what happened is okay.

This is not forgiveness. True forgiveness is not about the other person or the event. It's about setting ourselves free from the event that happened. Forgiveness is about *you*. It's self-forgiveness for everything you perceive that you've done wrong because of the trauma, because you have done *nothing* wrong. You have done the best you could under the circumstances you were given.

Forgiveness is about letting go of your self-judgments, self-criticism, and self-hatred. It's time. You can release them. The thoughts, feelings, and emotions that have ruled your life until this moment are no longer important. What matters is your capacity to forgive yourself, so that you can love yourself.

To be clear, forgiveness is not reconciliation with a perpetrator. The only way you reconcile with someone is if you consider it a valuable relationship. But there has to be some sort of contrition shown by the perpetrator, and they need to have demonstrated they are safe to be around.

Some people want their perpetrator to acknowledge what they did and to take responsibility for the harm they caused. But as psychologist Margaret Paul, Ph.D., explained, "We can't make them do that, no matter what we do. We have no control over whether somebody ever acknowledges that they were abusive. To focus on getting the abuser to take responsibility and admit it is to keep you stuck in the past."[6]

It's also very rare for a perpetrator to acknowledge what they've done. "With a child who has been traumatized by parents, the parents have so much dissociation they don't even know they did it, or if they know, they have so much shame there's no way they're going to admit they did it," Dr. Paul continued. "So, while it would be greatly healing if someone who abused you said, 'I'm sorry' and they take responsibility, it's really rare for that to happen."[7]

Instead, as we work toward compassion and forgiveness for ourselves, it opens the door to forgive our perpetrators. Not for what they did, but for their own imperfections, struggles, and pain. As your self-forgiveness grows, you see that the person who abused you was coming from their own deep level of trauma and woundedness.

Dr. Paul explained it like this: "People who abuse, they don't know what love is. They don't know what compassion is. They're deeply abandoning themselves. They're projecting all their self-loathing onto their child or others. Eventually, we get to understand that and to see that they were just coming from their own deep woundedness. And we can forgive. We don't forget, we don't condone, but it does mean that we're no longer blaming. We're no longer feeling like victims of whatever happened to us."[8]

And as we reach this place, we begin to soften toward others and their experiences being human, and that includes some of the people we have blamed for hurting us or who were responsible for the experience we endured.

How do we reach forgiveness? Sometimes it happens organically as you go through therapies. That's the case for many of Dr. Julie Brown Yau's patients. Rarely do they talk about forgiveness, but it naturally arises as they experience more compassion for themselves and this human journey that they're on.

Other times, the trauma experts we spoke to use practices to help their patients open that door. We're sharing some of the most profoundly moving ones here. Let's take a look.

Inner-Child Healing

As children, we experience a lot that we don't have the ability to process and understand. We also don't often have the same support that we do as adults, including self-nurturing practices, healers, friends, coaches, and therapists who can help us make sense of our experiences and reactions.

As kids, we make up our own stories and beliefs that we carry into adulthood but that don't serve our highest and greatest good. Part of our trauma work can be to forgive ourselves for what we have created and to help ourselves see the experience through a different lens.

Inner-child work can help us do that.

How it works is you start by checking in with your body. You notice an emotion you're feeling or tension or pain in a part of your body. Let's say you feel it in your gut. Then you'd ask yourself, *What does it feel like? What is its texture? What is its temperature?*

Questions like these move you out of your head, into your body, and then into where that trauma got stuck and stored. From there you'd ask, *How old does it [that pain or stuck energy] feel?* Usually a childhood age will immediately spring to mind.

Then you'd ask, *When do you remember feeling like that? When did you have that same feeling in your belly?*

A memory may form. For instance, say you remember being eight years old and standing in the hallway at school, staring at a picture you painted in art class that was hanging on the wall. You felt really uncomfortable, thinking kids were judging it and that it wasn't good enough.

In this memory, you—as your adult self—can go stand or sit next to yourself as an eight-year-old. You don't change the situation, but you adjust the way you relate to yourself at the time. As the adult, you may say to the child, "Hey, that is an awesome painting. I love it. You did a great job."

Your younger self will probably say, "No, that was really bad, and I don't agree with you. Who do you think you are? I think it looks ugly."

Then you respond by saying, "Really, you think that looks ugly, huh?"

"Yes, I do."

"Okay, well, why?"

You're having a dialogue with yourself and creating space to have an honest, open conversation about your thoughts and feelings—and ultimately beliefs. For every "negative" thought or emotion, you get to counter with a positive, life-affirming one. That alone, that cheerleading and support that you're giving to yourself, can create so much healing.

If you didn't feel loved or supported in that moment as a kid, you get to give that to yourself now as a wiser, older, more mature, and more nurturing human being. You don't change the past, but you get to change the love that surrounds it.

Many of the experts we talked to said that inner-child work can be one of the most powerful ways we can experience self-forgiveness. As a child, we may have bought into the belief that we weren't good enough, or we sucked, or we were ugly, but as an adult, returning to that moment and seeing our younger selves for what they went through, we get to say, "I forgive myself for having judged myself all of these years. Wow, I had no idea how hard I was on myself and still am. But I didn't do anything wrong. I did the best I could."

The key is that you're forgiving yourself for the judgment you've held on to for all of these years. You're letting go of the story, and you're giving yourself the support, encouragement, validation, respect, and love that you didn't receive in that moment.

This is powerful medicine, indeed.

Mirror Work

In 2013, Dr. Keesha Ewers, an integrative medicine expert, conducted a small pilot study of 100 women called the HURT Study (healing unresolved trauma). She wanted to understand a recurring pattern that she saw in her new patients. Many came in asking for bioidentical hormone replacement therapy and other supplements. When she would ask why they needed them, almost without fail she'd hear about how their libido was gone (many were also exhausted and had brain fog).

As a follow-up, Dr. Ewers would ask them when the last time was that they had a libido or energy, or felt clear-headed. Often her patients responded with tears and shaky answers of "never." Other times, she'd get answers about how her patient's husband or wife had an affair five years ago. They had forgiven them, but they still didn't want to have sex.

Dr. Ewer's answer to her patients was the same—hormones will not fix the problem. If her patients wanted to fix their exhaustion, brain fog, weight gain, or hormone imbalances, they needed to address their undercurrent of trauma. Through her HURT study, Dr. Ewers discovered that to resolve the trauma, her patients had to have a willingness to *self-confront*. They had to be willing to look at whatever trauma happened in their lives and ask themselves, *Where can I take responsibility for this? Where in my life can I see that I'm attracting similar kinds of people or experiences, and why could that be? What is it that I need to adjust?*

From there it can take going through a trauma-release therapy, such as EMDR, cognitive behavioral therapy, or somatic experiencing—whatever treatment is right for them—and then eventually getting to forgiveness.

"I know people aren't going to want to hear about forgiveness, but it is not lip service," Dr. Ewers told us. "It's not, 'Oh, I forgive them.' There's actually a process I take people through that changes the brain, hormones, and the way the genetics are expressed. It's hard work, and you don't go from A to Z. You have to digest your feelings and experiences the same way you digest your food."[9]

In her HURT Study, forgiveness intervention was the only therapy Dr. Ewers used with women who had low libido and who had experienced trauma in their pasts. She didn't give them hormones or supplements, only her forgiveness exercise.

As she explained, it's not an easy one. According to Dr. Ewers, in our lives, we have all been both a victim and a perpetrator. All of us have hurt somebody. "When we are victimized, it's a very dysfunctional place of power to be in. People will say, 'I would never do that.' When we say that, we put ourselves into the space of righteous superiority and judging the person that hurt us. That puts us in a place where it makes us feel safe, like there's a boundary and a separation between us and them."[10]

Dr. Ewers used herself as an example of how her forgiveness exercise works. Dr. Ewers had been sexually abused by a person in authority when she was growing up. In her forgiveness exercise, she looked at the ego characteristics, or personality traits, of her perpetrator that she hated. She identified egomaniacal, misuse of power, and cruelty.

Then she used him and those traits as a mirror to herself and asked the question, "How did I use these personality traits in my life?"

"Every human has the same personality characteristics, but we use them differently," she explained. "We're all egomaniacal, we all misuse power, we're all cruel at some point, and we are also loving, compassionate, and kind. When I looked for a misuse of power, I said,

'Well, my gosh, I'm the parent of four children. I misused power all the time. I guilt tripped my son last week. That's a misuse of power.

"Then cruelty, and I said the same thing. I've definitely had moments in my parenting where I haven't been the kindest. Then egomaniacal. Well, yes, I've definitely led with my ego before in my life, and I could count on one hand and in under five seconds ways of doing that. While I wouldn't sexually abuse a child, I had done these other things. That's what is so difficult for people, because they look at the behavior, they want to say, 'I would never do that.'"[11]

In Dr. Ewers's mirror exercise, the idea is the perpetrator who hurt you is actually a teacher. They're showing you the personality traits that you dislike, hate, or despise in yourself. It doesn't mean that you are exhibiting them the same way or that you ever would. It's certainly not giving them a pass for what they did to you either.

It's showing you what it feels like to be on both sides, and it gives you the opportunity to be more mindful about your behaviors. "You get to feel, 'Oh, this is what it feels like to be on the receiving end when I do it, and then you get to say, 'I'm going to be watchful of that in myself now, and I'm going to change that behavior,'" said Dr. Ewers.[12]

This is forgiveness. It's making peace with ourselves for how we've shown up and treated others in the world—including how we've treated ourselves—and then it's making the conscious decision to act differently. This is truly transformative. How incredible is it that this kind of awakening comes from one of the darkest experiences in our lives?

Walking through Grief to Reach Forgiveness

Dr. Joan Rosenberg, a professor of graduate psychology at Pepperdine University, talked about how just saying "I forgive" doesn't work with individual and collective trauma. We have to make sense of how the experience impacted and changed our lives. This is true whether we survived a childhood or recent collective trauma.

To get to forgiveness, Dr. Rosenberg said that we need to *grieve* and that many of us live with *disguised grief*, where we've never allowed ourselves to feel, mourn, and move through the loss of something caused by an experience.

Dr. Rosenberg said there are signal words that she watches for that tell her disguised grief lies within someone, and they include indications of feeling bitter, resentful, cynical, pessimistic, and holding grudges. When we have these emotions swirling, we're living in a nonforgiving emotional state that doesn't allow us to lead a more loving, free, kind, or fuller life.

To reach forgiveness, we have to allow ourselves to grieve in different forms. Let's look at some of the expressions of grief.

Grieving over what you've gotten and didn't deserve. Think of all the bad stuff—the chaotic family home, alcoholic or drug-addicted parents, feeling in danger, physical assault or abuse, domestic violence, sexual assault, sexual violence, sexual abuse, emotional abuse. All of these kinds of abuse are neglect and would fall into the category of grieving over what we got and didn't deserve.

Grieving over what never was, and what we deserved and didn't get. This is about the missed opportunities and what we never received. It's the praise and the encouragement, the support, love, and affection in our early years. It's the job well done when we come home with good grades, the encouragement to go out and try something new even if it didn't turn out well, or somebody showing up for ball games or piano recitals. It's what the trauma derailed or left out from our lives.

Grieving over what is not now. It's what our lives look like today. It's facing the facts of our lives and acknowledging that maybe we're not exactly where we want to be or who we want to be.

Grieving over what may never be or someone who may never show up for us the way we longed for. This is about coming to grips with unfulfilled expectations and unmet needs and realizing that someone important to you—a parent, a spouse, a sibling—wasn't there for you or in the way you needed them to be at some time, and that may always be the case. It's grieving over that loss.

As we allow ourselves to feel every emotion that disguised grief is covering—pain, loss, separation, fear, loneliness—then we can start to make sense of the meaning that those "Big T" or "Little t" traumas had on us over time.

As Dr. Rosenberg explained, when you can allow yourself to grieve and move through it, then you can extract the impact and meaning those traumas have had on you. For example, a child who grew up in a chaotic home environment may have spent more time at school or studying as a way to escape and fend off the pain and chaos at home. All that time and focus on school helped them develop excellent academic skills and discipline, which in turn, granted them more opportunities to go further in life. The involvement in school would not have come about had it not been for their chaotic home life, and so they can extract a good, meaningful takeaway from a painful experience.

When we can find meaning from our traumas, then we can move into a forgiving space. Again, it's not about forgiving what happened; it's making peace that it did. You can't change the past, and you had no control over it. But you did turn it into something positive that affected you, changed you, and shaped you and the course of your life.

From here, we can start to let go of the past, because we've extracted the gold from it. Now you can let the rest of the trauma remain behind you.[13]

THE ROAD TO RECOVERY

One day while lying in bed, Jenny realized she had two options.

She could continue thinking the scary thoughts that she'd never get better and this was going to be as good as it got, or she could try forgiving herself for these thoughts, her emotions, and the stories she had created about how her life would turn out.

If I can forgive myself, then maybe I can start anew, she thought.

This meant accepting where she was in the moment and giving herself permission to acknowledge her needs and set boundaries around her energy and time, so she could heal—in the mind and body. She started very basic. If she needed water, she got a glass of water and would focus on drinking it. If she needed to lie down, she crawled into bed and focused on how soft the blankets and pillow felt.

She also stopped beating herself up for not hosting playdates and dinner parties. She stopped saying yes to all the volunteer requests.

Saying no was tough, but for Jenny, when she said no to someone else, she was saying yes to herself. And she started thanking her body and feeling grateful to it for keeping her safe by storing toxins in fat.

Once Jenny began forgiving herself and setting boundaries every day, she was able to slowly heal her physical ailments by reducing inflammation in her body. It took time and included adopting an anti-inflammatory diet. She removed sugar and alcohol first, finding healthier yet still tasty substitutes like raw honey. In two weeks, she noticed a difference. Then she removed cow's milk, refined oils, and GMOs. She upped her water intake too.

Later, she connected with nature to help her feel grounded, and she used supplements and homeopathic remedies. Over time, meditation returned to Jenny's self-care practice. She used a guided form that helped direct her overactive mind. This meditation, combined with reducing the inflammation and spending time outdoors, helped calm her nervous system.

From there the positive thoughts and affirmations followed.

Throughout this experience, Jenny realized it was the thoughts and stories she had made up about her physical experience that had caused so much damage and trauma in her life. Yes, she had to take specific actions to heal her body—it wasn't going to magically get better with her thoughts alone. But it was the combination that led to her recovery.

She's still working through her trauma. Today, she's trying to reteach her body that it's okay to let go of the extra weight. She can feel the fear that still resides, but she recognizes it and is willing to meet her body where it is—forgiving and giving it what it needs in each moment.

This is the ultimate lesson for all of us, because it's all any of us can do. We have to meet ourselves where we are today. Like Jenny, releasing our traumas requires constant acceptance and forgiveness. It's surrendering to where we find ourselves in life, letting go of judging ourselves for the role we've played, and ultimately grabbing the reins of responsibility for what is in our control and then working from there to unwind our pain.

Jenny shows us the power of forgiveness and self-love, which is available to you right now. It costs nothing. No matter where you are on your journey to releasing trauma, you can forgive yourself. You can start to set healthy boundaries like Jenny did. You may need to practice this regularly, but if you do, eventually it will become natural for you. Over time, your needs will change, just like Jenny's, but the more you gift yourself forgiveness now, the easier it will be for you to realize what you need.

REFLECTIONS

What feels right to you in this chapter? Do you notice a sensation of relief? Do any topics trigger tears? Give yourself a few moments to go inward and see what arises for you. Maybe you found yourself moved by setting healthy boundaries, practicing self-awareness, knowing your values, wall work, and building your "no" muscle. Maybe the idea of forgiveness hit a nerve and you want to try inner-child healing, mirror work, or walking through grief. Maybe the entire chapter resonated! You want to pay attention to anything that makes a strong impression. That's usually a sign that you've discovered an area that needs attention. If something does come up, ask yourself if it's something you want or need right now or if it's something to try later.

SAGE WISDOM

"Ultimately, what heals trauma is loving. You learn to love this thing that happened to you. You don't have to like that it happened, but you learn to wrap your loving around the horror, hurt, devastation."
—Dr. Lin Morel

CHAPTER 11

FREEDOM

Patricia thought she was going crazy.

It had started when her 18-year-old son had come to live with her. She had given birth to him when she was only 16. For the first nine months of his life, she had cared for him. But then the bishop in her Mormon church told her God had sent him a vision that her child should no longer be on earth with her. Maybe at one point, he'd know her as his mother, but now wasn't the time.

Patricia didn't want to give up her son, but then again, it was the leader of her church, a person of power and authority. She had been taught his word was law, so she put aside what she wanted and felt was right, and she agreed to the adoption.

For the next 18 years, Patricia threw herself into work and perfectionism. She started and grew successful multimillion-dollar businesses. She owned and operated a nationally recognized and award-winning exclusive boutique spa in Utah that was eventually acquired. If you met Patricia, on the outside, she looked like she had everything put together, the picture-perfect image of being fit and healthy and successful.

Not once did she tell anyone about her son. She carried so much shame and embarrassment. According to her faith, Patricia was wrong and had sinned when she got pregnant. For almost two decades, she had buried her trauma, trying her best to forget all about the son she gave birth to and gave up for adoption. But then her son came home. Sitting across from him in her living room, she couldn't ignore the pain, and seeing him had cracked open something deeper and darker within her.

Every night, her dreams were filled with horrifying images of her as a child being beaten, sexually abused, and shaken so violently that she would pass out. They were so disturbing that she drank and popped pills to numb herself.

But the dreams kept coming. At 40 years old, she didn't understand what was happening to her. One night, it got so intense that she fell to her knees in her bedroom and for the first time prayed to God to take her life or show her a path to healing.

The thought came that she should call a trauma center, so at 2 A.M., she did. Call it serendipity, luck, or divine intervention, but someone answered one of her calls, and they happened to have a bed available. "I'm coming," Patricia told them.

In the early-morning hours, before daylight even broke, she checked herself in and from there began the slow and excruciating process of unpacking the terrible truth that she had suppressed. For 13 years, Patricia had endured extreme physical, sexual, and emotional abuse at the hands of her family.

Resolving this deep pain did not come easily.

Once she was out of treatment, she often thought, *Oh my God, who will love me now? How will I ever meet someone who could love me knowing what had happened to me? What will people think of me now?*

The shame and fear were almost too much for Patricia to take. She wondered, *How do I die?* But the pull for life was equally strong, and in her darkest moments, she would ask the Universe for a way to be open to healing.

Again, she was given an answer in a dream: plant medicine.

On blind faith, Patricia ventured into the Costa Rican jungle to experience an iboga ceremony, which uses a psychedelic plant. It took her on a brutal journey into her past that took days to complete. She wasn't prepared for so many repressed memories to become unblocked, but now her life made sense in a way it hadn't before.

This one experience would become the gateway for deep, profound healing that would change her life forever.

Patricia became very intentional with seeking treatments and support systems, including trauma and sexual abuse therapists. She eliminated caffeine and alcohol from her diet, and anything else that would get in the way of her processing and releasing all of this stored pain. She did meditation and yoga, and eventually earned a degree in spiritual psychology and became a shaman.

Patricia's road to recovery hasn't always been easy. Some days and nights have felt dark and heavy. Sometimes she lies in bed, crying and grieving for the childhood she wishes that she had, for the loss of being protected, and for not being loved and cherished the way a baby and young girl should have been.

But she's kept walking, even after life has presented her with more challenges. Recently, Patricia lost her older sister to a drug overdose. The day before her sister died, they talked about their shared secret for the first time. Like Patricia, her sister had been severely abused, and Patricia knows it took her sister's life.

Her sister's death became the catalyst for Patricia's next act in life. She's taken all her business acumen, all the years of healing she's been through, and today she's working to help other people change and heal their lives too.

"I'll be damned if I lose another loved one because we're not able to tell our stories or because we're not able to use our voices in a way for good," Patricia told us. "For me, there's something so powerful in being able to say, 'I'm an incest survivor, and I can go from surviving to thriving, and truly make a difference.' I have often thought that there is no way I was put on this earth to go through all that I went through if it wasn't for good in the end. I've surrendered. I ask, 'How can I be of service? What can I do to give back? Let me transform all that I've been through and be a voice for those that don't have the courage to speak their truth yet.'"[1]

As Patricia has shared her story, she's been shocked by the magnitude of people who have survived sexual and physical abuse too. They have fueled her to keep walking her road to recovery and talking about her truth.

"I often think I can't believe I'm still living," she told us. "I can't believe I made it through that. I made it to the other side, and it is possible. Not only did I endure sexual abuse; it was physical, it was emotional, and it was being detached from my child—it was almost as if he died. This journey has been one of the most powerful, hard, gut wrenching, yet beautiful experiences of my life. Not easy, but beautiful."[2]

THE WORLD NEEDS YOU

When we first heard Patricia's story, it broke our hearts. We felt angry for what she and so many people have gone through in this world. But her story also reminds us that we always have the power to choose what we do with our lives, our time, and the trauma we've endured.

Our traumas do not define us. They help shape who we become. We have control over that. Patricia filled us with so much hope and inspiration. She's an incredibly strong, resourceful, brave soul who has lived through hell, yet she's *thriving*. Anyone who has the privilege of spending time with her can feel and see the inner light that shines from within.

She shares that with the world, and she's taken her pain and transformed it into something that can help others on their journeys to acceptance, self-love, self-forgiveness, and healing. Everyone who you met in this book has taken their pain, released it, and created something beautiful from it.

No matter what trauma you've endured, how long you've carried it, or how deeply embedded it is inside you, you can free yourself from the pain and suffering. Sometimes it is hard, and it takes work, determination, persistence, and a lot of self-forgiveness, but it's possible.

When you release your trauma, you unlock your inner light and radiance, and everywhere you go and everyone you meet feels it. You change the course of everyone's lives just by being you.

And now, more than ever, the world needs you. It needs your light.

It's selfish for us to say this, we know. Ultimately, each of us has to heal and resolve our traumas for ourselves. Yet we don't create this world and our experience of being human alone. It's co-created with everyone.

Right now, there is so much pain and suffering. We don't think it's a coincidence that we're facing some of the most monumental political, economic, environmental, and social challenges in history.

If we want a different future for the world—for our children and loved ones—then it starts with each of us, going in, facing the pain, and learning how to integrate it. Releasing that trapped pain leaves us feeling love and forgiveness. Imagine the individual and collective world we'd co-create if more people acted from this state of being?

We need as many people as possible to wake up and say, "No more. No longer will I live with this pain and torment. No longer will I suffer from my traumas. No longer will I allow myself to make decisions and take actions from that pain. I will heal. I will resolve this trauma, no matter how long it takes, no matter how many stops on this journey I make. I choose to heal. I choose to release my pain."

Patricia chose this path, and she keeps choosing it every day, no matter how hard or dark some days and nights still are. Everyone you met in these pages made the same choice.

Now it's your turn. You hold the power to change your life for the better, and in doing so, you change the world.

But it starts with you saying yes.

Yes, I am willing to have a different experience of life.

Yes, I am willing to go on this journey.

Yes, I am willing to release the pain.

Yes, I am willing to free myself from my trauma.

All of this is possible. We have listened in awe (and yes, sometimes tears) to countless stories of people just like you who have faced their inner shadows and have recovered from their "Big T" and "Little t" traumas. With courage and conviction in their hearts, they have learned how to feel and finally release their stored pain.

That's how we know that you can do it too. No matter what trauma you have faced, you can do this. No matter what you encounter along this journey, please don't stop. Don't give up on yourself.

You can resolve your trauma and live a happier, healthier, more vibrant life.

You can help co-create a brighter world.

You can be free.

SAGE WISDOM

"It isn't until we bring our trauma and what's happened to us into the light that we have the opportunity to heal on a deep and meaningful level."

—Patricia Damon

ENDNOTES

Chapter 1

1. Stacie Aamon Yeldell, interview with the authors, January 24, 2020.

2. Benjet, et al., "The Epidemiology of Traumatic Event Exposure Worldwide: Results from the World Mental Health Survey Consortium," *Psychological Medicine* 46, no 2 (October 29, 2015): 327–343. https://doi.org/10.1017/s0033291715001981.

3. Dr. Patrick Gentempo, DC, interview with the authors, July 8, 2019.

4. Brandy Gillmore, interview with the authors, May 17, 2019.

5. Dr. Carl Totton, interview with the authors, August 20, 2019.

6. Ibid.

7. "What Is Posttraumatic Stress Disorder?" American Psychiatric Association, accessed April 27, 2020, https://www.psychiatry.org/patients-families/ptsd/what-is-ptsd.

8. Ibid.

9. Ibid.

10. Stewart, et al., "Challenging Child Behaviours Positively Predict Symptoms of Posttraumatic Stress Disorder in Parents of Children with Autism Spectrum Disorder and Rare Diseases," *Research in Autism Spectrum Disorders* 69 (January 2020). https://doi.org/10.1016/j.rasd.2019.101467.

11. "What Is Posttraumatic Stress Disorder?" American Psychiatric Association, accessed April 27, 2020, https://www.psychiatry.org/patients-families/ptsd/what-is-ptsd.

Chapter 2

1. Dr. Totton, interview.

2. Ibid.

3. Dr. Gentempo, interview.

4. Taylor Ross, interview with authors, February 6, 2020.

5. Ibid.

6. Gillmore, interview.

7. Ibid.

8. Mary Morrissey, interview with the authors, August 9, 2019.

9. Dr. Yvonne Farrell, interview with the authors, September 11, 2019.

10. Ibid.

11. "Traumatic Brain Injury Overview," Mayo Clinic, accessed May 5, 2020, https://www.mayoclinic.org/diseases-conditions/traumatic-brain-injury/symptoms-causes/syc-20378557.

12. Ibid.

13. Simon, et al., "The Far-Reaching Scope of Neuroinflammation after Traumatic Brain Injury," *Nature Reviews Neurology* 13 (February 10, 2017): 171–191. https://doi.org/10.1038/nrneurol.2017.13.

Chapter 3

1. Rick Nauert, "Psychological Trauma Tied to Irritable Bowel Syndrome," Psych Central, last updated August 8, 2018, https://psychcentral.com/news/2011/11/01/psychological-trauma-tied-to-irritable-bowel-syndrome/30933.html.

2. Dr. Jorina Elbers, interview with the authors, November 14, 2019.

3. Dube, et al., "Cumulative Childhood Stress and Autoimmune Diseases in Adults," *Psychosomatic Medicine* 71, no 2 (February–March 2009): 243–250. https://doi.org/10.1097/PSY.0b013e3181907888.

4. Kirsten Schultz, "Are Childhood Trauma and Chronic Illness Connected?" *Healthline*, https://www.healthline.com/health/chronic-illness/childhood-trauma-connected-chronic-illness#Whats-next?.

5. Odelya Gertel Kraybill, "PTSD May Be a Risk Factor for Autoimmune Disease," *Psychology Today*, February 28, 2020, https://www.psychologytoday.com/us/blog/expressive-trauma-integration/202002/ptsd-may-be-risk-factor-autoimmune-disease.

6. Keiko Iguchi, "Boosting Immunity Through Gut Bacteria," *Newsweek*, February 22, 2019, https://www.newsweek.com/gut-bacteria-immune-system-probiotics-1333541.

7. "Past Trauma May Haunt Your Future Health," *Harvard Health Publishing*, February 2019, https://www.health.harvard.edu/diseases-and-conditions/past-trauma-may-haunt-your-future-health.

8. Ibid.

9. Dr. Keesha Ewers, interview with the authors, August 9, 2019.

10. Breit, et al., "Vagus Nerve as Modulator of the Brain–Gut Axis in Psychiatric and Inflammatory Disorders," *Frontiers in Psychiatry* 9, no. 44 (March 13, 2018). https://doi.org/10.3389/fpsyt.2018.00044.

11. Ibid.

12. Ibid.

13. "Obesity and Overweight," Centers for Disease Control and Prevention, accessed May 15, 2020, https://www.cdc.gov/nchs/fastats/obesity-overweight.htm.

14. Marc David, interview with the authors, June 27, 2019.

15. Ibid.

16. Marc David, interview.

17. Ibid.

Chapter 4

1. Association for Psychological Science, "Can Fetus Sense Mother's Psychological State? Study Suggests Yes," *ScienceDaily*, last updated November 10, 2011, www.sciencedaily.com/releases/2011/11/111110142352.htm.

2. Dr. Joanne Barron, interview with the authors, February 6, 2020.

3. Dave Richo, interview with the authors, November 12, 2019.

4. Ibid.

5. Jeff Ball, interview with the authors, January 23, 2020.

6. Ibid.

Chapter 5

1. Gilad Hirschberger, "Collective Trauma and the Social Construction of Meaning," *Frontiers in Psychology* 9, no 1441 (August 10, 2018). https://doi.org/10.3389/fpsyg.2018.01441.

2. Alex Hern, "Revealed: Catastrophic Effects of Working as a Facebook Moderator," *The Guardian*, September 17, 2019, https://www.theguardian.com/technology/2019/sep/17/revealed-catastrophic-effects-working-facebook-moderator.

3. Ibid.

4. Stacie Aamon Yeldell, interview with the authors, January 24, 2020.

5. Mohatt, et al., "Historical Trauma as Public Narrative: A Conceptual Review of How History Impacts Present-Day Health," *Social Science & Medicine* 106 (April 2014): 128–136. https://doi.org/10.1016/j.socscimed.2014.01.043.

6. Smith College, "Dr. Maria Yellow Horse Brave Heart Speaks on Historical Trauma," accessed May 15, 2020, https://ssw.smith.edu/about/news-events/dr-maria-yellow-horse-brave-heart-returns-smith-give-rapoport-lecture.

7. Ibid.

8. Ibid.

9. Ibid.

10. Gwen Dittmar, interview with the authors, September 11, 2019.

11. Ibid.

12. "Suicide: One Person Dies Every 40 Seconds," World Health Organization, press release, September 9, 2019, https://www.who.int/news-room/detail/09-09-2019 -suicide-one-person-dies-every-40-seconds.

13. Ibid.

14. Ibid.

15. "Suicide Rising Across the US," Centers for Disease Control, accessed May 28, 2020, https://www.cdc.gov/vitalsigns/suicide/index.html.

16. Dr. Sam Rader, interview with the authors, August 20, 2019.

17. Ibid.

18. Dr. Mark L. Gordon, interview with authors, September 18, 2020.

19. Laura Santhanam, "Youth Suicide Rates Are on the Rise in the U.S.," *PBS News Hour*, October 18, 2019, https://www.pbs.org/newshour/health/youth-suicide -rates-are-on-the-rise-in-the-u-s.

20. Ibid.

21. Ibid.

Chapter 6

1. Arielle Hanien, interview with the authors, February 19, 2020.

2. Ibid.

3. Dr. Ruchira Densert, interview with the authors, February 6, 2020.

4. Dr. Debi Silber, interview with the authors, August 8, 2019.

5. Margaret Paul, interview with the authors, August 10, 2019.

6. Sarvada Chandra Tiwari, "Loneliness: A Disease?" *Indian Journal of Psychiatry* 55, no 4, (2013): 320–322. https://doi.org/10.4103/0019-5545.120536.

7. Dr. Patrick Gentempo, interview.

8. Ibid.

Chapter 7

1. Dr. Keesha Ewers, interview.

2. Dr. Carl Totton, interview.

3. Ibid.

4. Dr. Sam Rader, interview.

5. Ibid.

6. William Hufschmidt, interview with the authors, February 2, 2020.

7.   Stephanie Speights, interview with the authors, September 12, 2019.

8.   William Hufschmidt, interview.

9.   Dr. Sam Rader, interview.

10. Dr. Sam Rader, interview.

11. Dr. Sam Rader, interview.

12. Dr. Carl Totton, interview.

13. Ibid.

14. Dr. Lin Morel, interview with the authors, July 15, 2019.

15. Ibid.

16. Darcy Lubbers, interview with the authors, January 24, 2020.

17. Ibid.

18. Stacie Aamon Yeldell, interview.

19. Stacie Aamon Yeldell, interview.

20. Stacie Aamon Yeldell, interview.

21. Gabrielle Kaufman, interview with the authors, January 23, 2020.

22. Gabrielle Kaufman, interview.

Chapter 8

1.   Dr. Keesha Ewers, interview with the authors, August 8, 2019.

2.   Dr. Mark L. Gordon, interview.

3.   Dr. Mark L. Gordon, interview.

4.   "Organic Foods: Are They Safer? More Nutritious?" Mayo Clinic, accessed June 1, 2020, https://www.mayoclinic.org/healthy-lifestyle/nutrition-and-healthy -eating/in-depth/organic-food/art-20043880.

5.   Yasmin Anwar, "Nature is proving to be awesome medicine for PTSD," UC Berkeley News, July 12, 2018, https://news.berkeley.edu/2018/07/12/awe-nature -ptsd/.

6.   Hon K. Yuen and Gavin R. Jenkins, "Factors Associated with Changes in Subjective Well-Being Immediately After Urban Park Visit," *International Journal of Environmental Health Research* 30, no 2 (February 13, 2019): 134–145. https:// doi.org/10.1080/09603123.2019.1577368.

7.   Dr. Carl Totton, interview.

8.   Dr. Mark L. Gordon, interview.

9.   Krediet, et al., "Reviewing the Potential of Psychedelics for the Treatment of PTSD," *International Journal of Neuropsychopharmacology* 23, no 6 (June 2020): 385–400. https://doi.org/10.1093/ijnp/pyaa018.

10. Ibid.

11. Ibid.

12. Arielle Hanien, interview.

13. Ibid.

14. Andrew Marr, interview with the authors, October 29, 2019.

Chapter 9

1. Jodi Cohen, interview with the authors, August 8, 2019.

2. Ibid.

3. Ibid.

4. Stephanie Speights, interview with the authors, September 12, 2019.

5. Ibid.

6. Darcy Lubbers, interview with the authors, January 24, 2020.

7. Dr. Patrick Gentempo, interview.

Chapter 10

1. Dr. Yvonne Farrell, interview.

2. Ibid.

3. Dr. Sam Rader, interview.

4. Ibid.

5. Ibid.

6. Margaret Paul, interview.

7. Ibid.

8. Ibid.

9. Dr. Keesha Ewers, interview.

10. Ibid.

11. Ibid.

12. Ibid.

13. Dr. Joan Rosenberg, interview with the authors, August 8, 2019.

Chapter 11

1. Patricia Damon, interview with the authors, July 16, 2019.

2. Ibid.

INDEX

A

abandonment, childhood trauma and, 58
abuse, types of, 56–60
Academy for Integrative Medicine, 38
acceptance ("The Five Basic Needs"),
    55–56
ACE. *See* adverse childhood experiences
acupuncture points, 108
addiction
    childhood trauma and, 57
    intergenerational trauma and, 70
    mind and body connection, 21, 27–28
    story about trauma and recovery from,
        81–82, 92–93
adverse childhood experiences (ACE). *See
    also* childhood trauma
    ACE Quiz, 13
    ACE Study (Centers for Disease
        Control and Prevention, Kaiser
        Permanente), 37–38
    gut health and, 37–38
affection ("The Five Basic Needs"), 55–56
affirmation, 147–149
alcohol, eliminating, 123. *See also*
    addiction
"alley up" gatherings, 144–145
allowing ("The Five Basic Needs"), 55–56
American Psychiatric Association, 11
amygdala, 20–21, 23, 39
ancient traditions and natural remedies,
    117–134
    for biochemistry in balance, 121–122
    diet and nutrition, 122–123
    meditation and, 126–128
    Mother Nature and, 124–126
    movement and, 123–124
    plant medicine and, 128–129
    Reflection exercise, 133
    sacred rituals and ceremonies, 129–131

Sage Wisdom about, 134
shamans, 71, 177
stories of trauma and recovery, 117–
    118, 131–133
stressors of modern-day life, 119–121
anger, childhood trauma of, 59
appreciation ("The Five Basic Needs"),
    55–56
art, as self-nurturing practice, 139–142,
    146–147
art therapy, 109–110
attention ("The Five Basic Needs"), 55–56
autoimmune diseases, 37–38
Ayurvedic medicine, 122–123

B

Barron, Joanne, 45
"Big T" traumas
    of childhood, 48–49
    defined, 7
    importance of all types of trauma, 10
    meditation for, 127
    symptoms of, 12–13
    therapy for, 98, 101, 106, 109 (*see also*
        therapy)
biochemistry in balance, 121–122
birth and parenting. *See* childhood
    trauma
body fat. *See* weight
bodywork, 102–104
bonding in early infancy, 51–52
boundaries
    as essential, 155
    saying "no" and, 157, 162–163
    self-awareness for, 158–159
    setting healthy boundaries, 156–158
    values and, 159–161
    Wall Work for, 161–162

with creativity and arts, 139–142
finding community for, 143–145
finding your unique activities for,
141–142
for physical pain from trauma, 31
Reflection exercise, 151
Sage Wisdom about, 151
for self-care, 136–139
self-talk and, 147–149
stories about trauma and recovery,
135–136, 149–150
serotonin, 36
sexual abuse, childhood trauma of, 57
shamans, 71, 177
Shojai, Pedram
background of, xiv, xx–xxi
Exhausted, xv, xvii, 41
Silber, Debi, 88–89
snap, stop, notice, and pause technique,
101
social media, 75–76
societal trauma, 65–79
as collective trauma, 66–67
fear-based media and entertainment,
68–69
historical trauma, 71–73
intergenerational trauma, 69–71
Reflection exercise, 79
Sage Wisdom about, 79
stories about trauma and recovery,
65–66, 76–79
suicide and, 73–76
somatic therapy, 105–106, 161–162
Speights, Stephanie, 102–103, 144–145
spirituality. *See also* ancient traditions
and natural remedies; spiritual trauma
building spiritual community, 145–
147
creativity/arts vs. religious practice,
147
spiritual trauma, 81–94
connection needs, 82–83, 85, 90–91
false beliefs and, 86–89
finding purpose and, 90–91
Islamic people, prejudice against, 73
Reflection exercise, 93–94
religion as source of trauma, 82–84
rewriting spiritual story for, 89–90
Sage Wisdom about, 94
stories about trauma and recovery,
81–82, 92–93
trust and faith needs, 84–86
stomach pain. *See* gut health
stories about trauma and recovery

ancient traditions and natural
remedies, 117–118, 131–133
childhood trauma, 47, 61–62
freedom from trauma, 175–179
gut health, 33, 43–44
mind and body connection, 17–18,
24–25, 30–32
seeking therapy and, 97–98, 113–115
self-nurturing practices, 135–136,
149–150
societal trauma, 65–66, 76–79
spiritual trauma, 81–82, 92–93
trauma, 3–4, 14–15
stress, chronic, 8, 34, 38, 47, 62, 153. *See
also* trauma
suicide, 73–76, 88
sympathetic nervous system, 20–21

T

tai chi, 123–124
Taoist Institute, 9
tapping (thought field therapy,
Emotional Freedom Technique),
107–108
therapy, 97–115. *See also* ancient
traditions and natural remedies;
forgiveness; self-nurturing practices;
stories about trauma and recovery
for the body, 102–104
for childhood trauma, 54
cognitive behavioral therapy, 14,
100–101
common and effective therapies,
overview, 98–99
emotional freedom technique
(tapping), 107–108
expressive arts therapy, 108–113
eye movement desensitization
reprogramming (EMDR), 14,
106–107
finding trauma-informed therapists,
99
intergenerational trauma and, 70
for the mind, 100–102
for the mind-body connection,
104–106
psychoanalytic therapy, 15, 101–102
Reflection exercise for seeking therapy,
115
Sage Wisdom about, 115
somatic therapy, 105–106, 161–162

ACKNOWLEDGMENTS

Writing a book is no small undertaking. Thankfully, we had help from an extraordinary group of people. First, our deepest thanks to our contributors: Fumiko Takatsu, Brandy Gillmore, Marc David, Patrick Gentempo, Lin Morel, Harry Adelson, Patricia Damon, Joan Rosenberg, Debi Silber, Jodi Cohen, Sandra Scheinbaum, Mary Morrissey, Keesha Ewers, Cassie Bjork, Bree Argetsinger, Margaret Paul, Sarah Rattray, Terry Wahls, Titus Chiu, Natasha Fallahi, Bita Yadidi, Mindy Gorman-Plutzer, Sam Rader, Carl Totton, Michael Mollura, Udo Erasmus, Garry Lineham, Gwen Dittmar, Yvonne Farrell, Hank Lutz, Julie Brown Yau, Stephanie Speights, Mark Gordon, Andrew Marr, Sarah Nannen, Taylor Ross, Adriana Marchione, Linda Chrisman, Jorina Elbers, Jamie McHugh, Laura Kleinman, James Gordon, Kevin Troiano, Jenny Carr, Jeff Ball, Gabrielle Kaufman, Stacie Aamon Yeldell, Catherine Scherwenka, Darcy Lubbers, Summer Lall, Laura Kalmes, Ruchira Densert, Joanne Barron, Roseann Capanna-Hodge, Sousan Abadian, Arielle Hanien, William Hufschmidt, Christian Gonzalez. *Thank you* for sharing your wisdom and inspiration with us.

Researching, organizing, shooting, and producing thousands of hours of footage is only possible with help. We are blessed to work with the best film and production crew in the business. Thank you to Lorenzo Phan, Mileen Patel, Courtney Donnelly, Sean Rivas, Carl Lindahl, and Dave Girtsman for sharing your energy, enthusiasm, and talent with us on this project.

On the book front, we are thankful to Amanda Ibey for her incredible ability to connect the dots between our vision, our contributors' wisdom, and our readers' struggles. Your skill, professionalism, and wordsmithing are unmatched. This is our second book together, and we're grateful for your partnership and collaboration. Courtney Donnelly, thank you for reviewing early drafts of this manuscript and for providing thoughtful feedback that elevated the book.

To Reid Tracy and Patty Gift at Hay House, *thank you* for trusting us, supporting us, and believing in us and this project. To Lisa Cheng, our editor, and the entire Hay House team, thank you for bringing your skills, wisdom, and excitement to this project. It is stronger because of all of you.

ABOUT THE AUTHORS

Dr. Pedram Shojai is a man with many titles. He is the founder of Well.org; the *New York Times* best-selling author of *The Urban Monk, Rise and Shine, The Art of Stopping Time,* and *Inner Alchemy*; and the co-author of *Exhausted*. He is the producer and director of the movies *Vitality, Origins,* and *Prosperity*. He has also produced several documentary series, including *Interconnected, Gateway to Health,* and *Exhausted*. In his spare time, he's a Taoist abbot, a doctor of Oriental medicine, a kung fu world traveler, a fierce global green warrior, an avid backpacker, a devout alchemist, a qigong master, and an old-school Jedi bio-hacker working to preserve our natural world and wake us up to our full potential. You can find him online at www.theurbanmonk.com.

Nick Polizzi is a producer and director of feature-length documentaries about holistic alternatives to conventional medicine. He is the founder of the Sacred Science, director of the feature documentary by the same name, and author of the book based on the film. He is also the co-author of *Exhausted*. Nick's mission as host and executive producer of the docuseries *Remedy: Ancient Medicines for Modern Illness* is to honor, preserve, and share powerful, evidence-based healing technologies with those who have been failed by modern medicine and the system as a whole. He has been traveling the world, documenting forgotten healing methods, ever since he cured himself of a debilitating illness at age 25 using a traditional therapy. You can visit him online at www.thesacredscience.com.

Hay House Titles of Related Interest

We hope you enjoyed this Hay House book. If you'd like to receive our online catalog featuring additional information on Hay House books and products, or if you'd like to find out more about the Hay Foundation, please contact:

Hay House, Inc., P.O. Box 5100, Carlsbad, CA 92018-5100
(760) 431-7695 or (800) 654-5126
(760) 431-6948 (fax) or (800) 650-5115 (fax)
www.hayhouse.com® • www.hayfoundation.org

———

Published in Australia by: Hay House Australia Pty. Ltd.,
18/36 Ralph St., Alexandria NSW 2015
Phone: 612-9669-4299 • *Fax:* 612-9669-4144
www.hayhouse.com.au

Published in the United Kingdom by: Hay House UK, Ltd.,
The Sixth Floor, Watson House, 54 Baker Street, London W1U 7BU
Phone: +44 (0)20 3927 7290 • *Fax:* +44 (0)20 3927 7291
www.hayhouse.co.uk

Published in India by: Hay House Publishers India,
Muskaan Complex, Plot No. 3, B-2, Vasant Kunj, New Delhi 110 070
Phone: 91-11-4176-1620 • *Fax:* 91-11-4176-1630
www.hayhouse.co.in

———

Access New Knowledge.
Anytime. Anywhere.

Learn and evolve at your own pace
with the world's leading experts.

www.hayhouseU.com

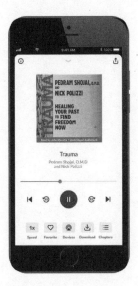